FOOD FOR THE FAST LANE

Recipes to Power your Body and Mind

DERVAL O'ROURKE

GILL & MACMILLAN

Gill & Macmillan
Hume Avenue
Park West
Dublin 12
www.gillmacmillanbooks.ie

978 07171 6288 8

Photography by Neil Hurley
Photos on pp. vi, x, xiv–xv, xxviii–xxix, xxxiii, 12–13, 114, 121, 172 and 178 by Karen Shinkins; photos on pp. 22 and 45 by Patrick Bolger;
photo on p. ix © INPHO/Dan Sheridan; photo on p. xx–xxi © PCN Photography/Alamy; photo on p. 82–83 © AFP/Getty Images; photo on
page 142–143 © Brendan Moran/Sportsfile
Food styling by Orla Neligan of Cornershop Productions
Assistant to stylist: Aga Wypych
Design by Fidelma Slattery
Edited by Dog's-ear
Indexed by Eileen O'Neill
Printed by Printer Trento Srl, Italy

PROPS
Avoca: HQ Kilmacanogue, Bray, Co. Wicklow. T: (01) 2746939; E: info@avoca.ie; www.avoca.ie
Meadows & Byrne: Dublin, Cork, Galway, Clare, Tipperary. T: (01) 2804554/(021) 4344100; E: info@meadowsandbyrne.ie;
www.meadowsandbyrne.com
Eden Home & Garden: 1–4 Temple Grove, Temple Road, Blackrock, Co. Dublin. T: (01) 7642004; edenhomeandgarden@hotmail.com;
www.edenhomeandgarden.ie
Article: Powerscourt Townhouse, South William Street, Dublin 2. T: (01) 6799268; E: items@articledublin.com; www.articledublin.com
House of Fraser: Dundrum Town Centre, Dublin 16. T: (01) 2991400; E: dundrum@hof.co.uk; www.houseoffraser.co.uk
Marks & Spencer: Dundrum Town Centre, Dundrum, Dublin 14. T: (01) 2991300; www.marksandspencer.com
Homebase: Nutgrove Retail Park, Nutgrove Ave, Dublin 14. T: (01) 4916118; www.homebase.co.uk
TK Maxx: The Park, Carrickmines, Dublin 18. T: (01) 2074798; www.tkmaxx.ie
Historic Interiors: Oberstown, Lusk, Co Dublin. T: (01) 8437174; E: killian@historicinteriors.net
Helen Turkington: 47 Dunville Avenue, Ranelagh, Dublin 6. T: 01 4125138; E: info@helenturkington.com; www.helenturkington.com

This book is typeset in Frutiger and Naïve.

The paper used in this book comes from the wood pulp of managed forests. For every tree felled, at least one tree is planted, thereby renewing natural resources.

A CIP catalogue record for this book is available from the British Library.

ACKNOWLEDGEMENTS

There are so many people that made this book a reality. I'm extremely grateful to everybody for their time and energy.

To my lovely husband, Peter, thank you for being a big part of this – for everything from recipe testing, to washing up, to encouraging me. You're a superstar.

My sister, Clodagh, has helped me with every aspect of this book. She has typed, tasted and tested every recipe at some stage. Thanks for being brill.

My parents, Eva and Terry, are great. My mum gets special thanks for doing lots of work at the food shoot.

My mother-in-law, Sally O'Leary, was a huge help – from cooking, to styling, to suggesting ideas. Thank you!

Emma Farrell and Ronan Vaughan from Dog's-ear made this idea into a book. Their passion, commitment and great sense of humour have been a joy to work with. *Merci!*

My great friend Declan Lee, thank you for making this happen all that time ago.

The days spent photographing the recipes for this book were so much fun thanks to the superb work of Orla Neligan and Neil Hurley. It was a pleasure! Thanks to Aga Wypych for assisting on this.

The stunning book design is Fidelma Slattery's great work. Thank you!

A big thank you to the crew at Gill & Macmillan for believing in this project and getting behind it. Deirdre Nolan, Teresa Daly and Catherine Gough, you've been great.

There are lots of pictures in this book that were taken by my talented photographer friend, Karen Shinkins. A big thank you to her for letting me use them.

My coaches, Sean and Terrie Cahill, have been a rock of support for me. No matter what it is I've been trying to achieve – from jumping hurdles to writing recipes – I could not have asked for two better people to work with. I feel privileged to have them in my corner. Thank you Team Cahill.

Martina McCarthy, I'll simply say thanks for always being you!

SOURCES OF INSPIRATION

Andrea Cullen has inspired so much of this book from the years I've spent working with her.

Lynda Booth and all the crew at Dublin Cookery School gave me such a great set of kitchen skills.

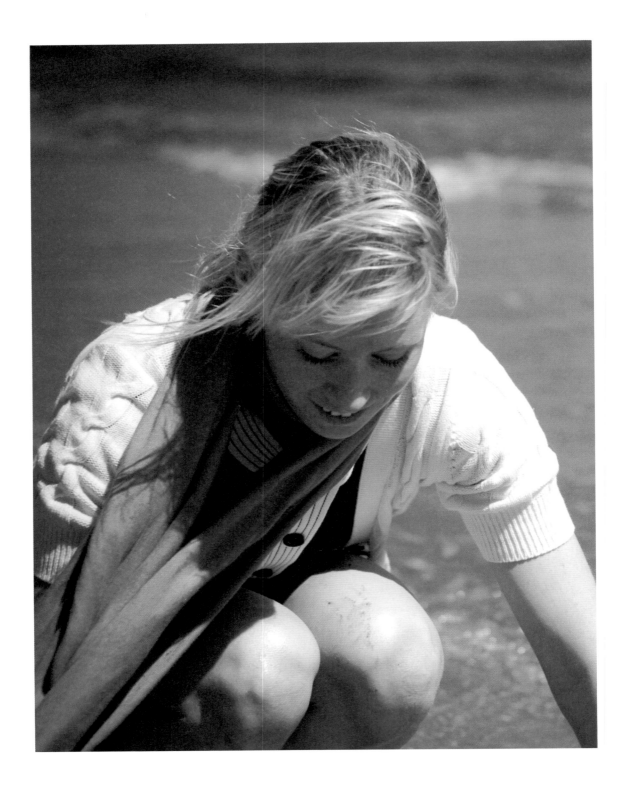

CONTENTS

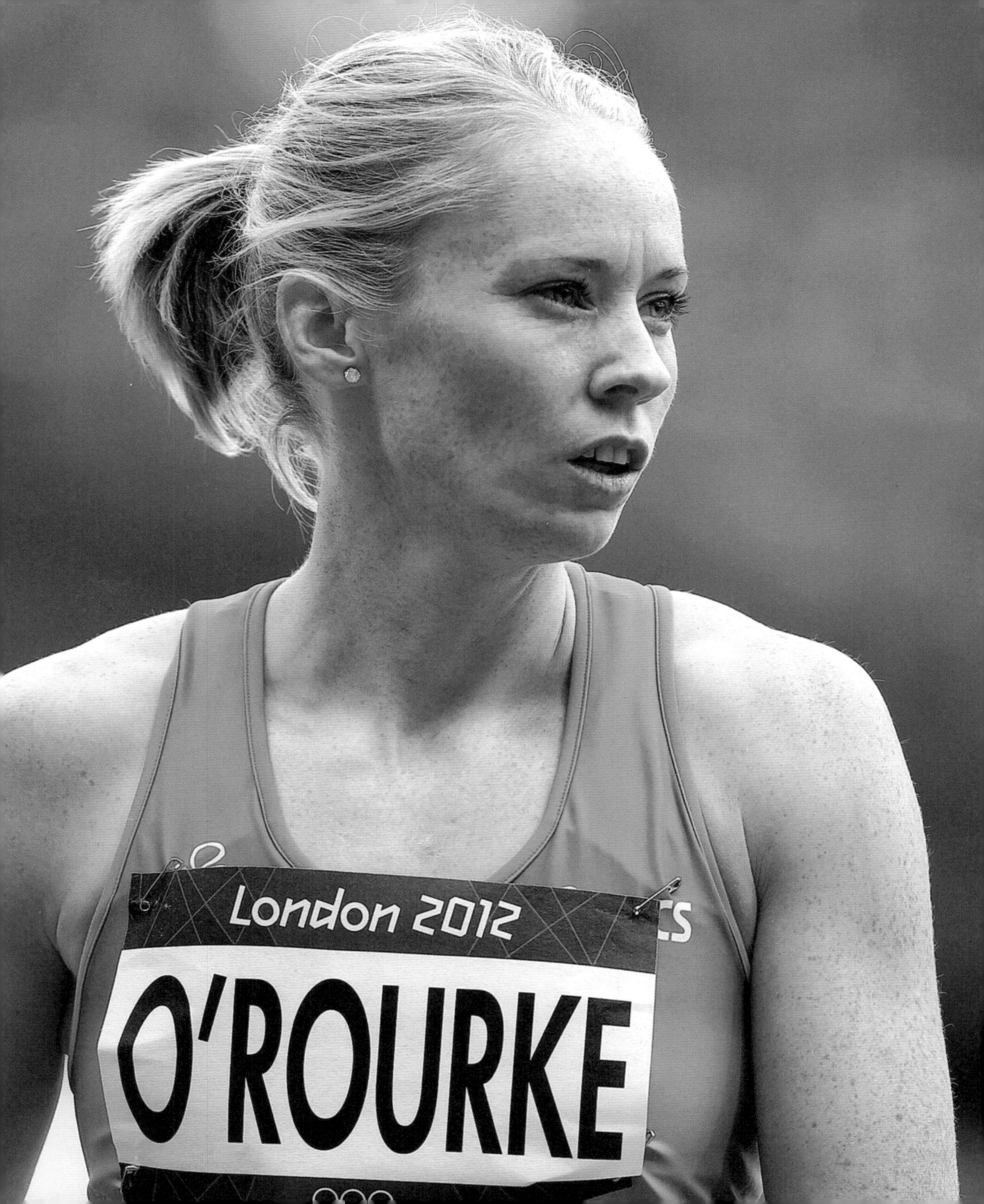
London 2012
O'ROURKE

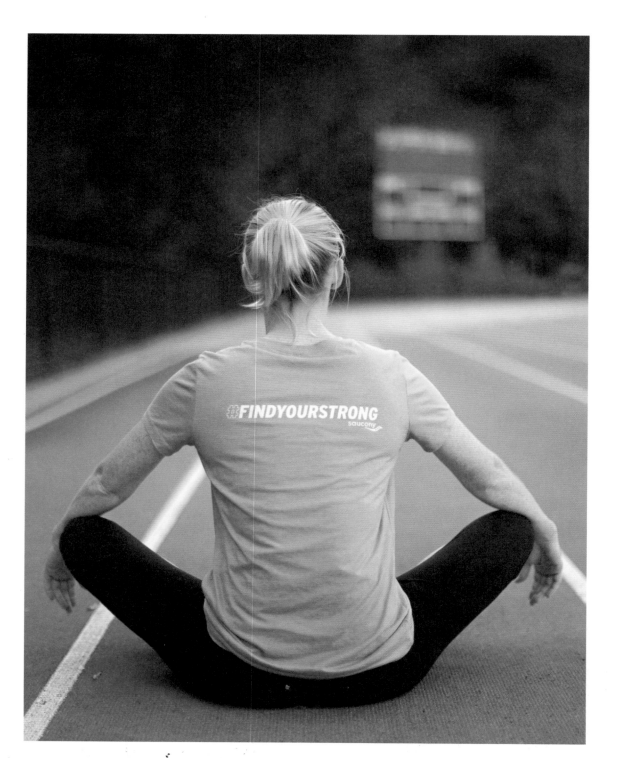

EVERYTHING IS INTERTWINED

Four weeks before the Olympic Games in Athens in 2004 I travelled to a race in Thessaloniki in Greece. I felt really sick during the journey but assumed that it wasn't anything serious. I checked into the hotel before midnight and tried to settle in and sleep for the night. I felt worse as the night wore on and it got to the stage where I was unable to walk or stand because my stomach cramps were so severe. At around six in the morning, I was rushed to hospital. I was diagnosed with severe food poisoning and appendicitis. If the doctors removed my appendix, it meant I would not have the opportunity to race at the Olympic Games.

The doctors treated me with antibiotics and kept me in hospital for six days. I was released and sent back to Ireland. I was 6kg lighter and in very bad health. The medical advice was to skip the Olympics and recover. But I wasn't willing to do that. The Olympics come once every four years. No athlete knows for sure if they will ever make an Olympics. And even when they do make one Olympics, they can never be sure what the next four years will bring and whether they will be good enough to even make the team.

I decided to go to Athens 2004. I lined up to race. I was 22 and one of the youngest members of the Irish Olympic team. It was one of the worst performances of my entire career and possibly had the biggest impact on my future running.

I trailed home in seventh place and I left the track feeling absolutely devastated. After the race, I hung around outside the stadium on my own. I could see the Olympic flame in the distance. I sat down and had a long think about things. I decided that if I was going to be an athlete, then I didn't want to be a bad one. Making a team would never be enough for me. I wanted to excel and to try to be one of the best in the world.

I kept thinking about my recent illness and my stay in hospital. I knew that being in hospital four weeks before the games had wiped any chance of me competing well. The message was loud and clear: I wasn't paying enough attention to my general health. I was depending solely on the work I was doing on the track and in the gym. And that was not enough.

xi

Sitting outside the Olympic Stadium in Greece was a wake-up call for me. From that point on, I changed as an athlete. I started to think about how everything in my life had a connection to my health and fitness. Everything is intertwined. If I wanted to achieve my ultimate performance goals, then I needed to make sure that I was paying attention to lots of things in my life. I needed to sleep better. I needed to eat better. I needed to live better. My college days were coming to an end. I was at a crossroads. I didn't want to waste my time coming up with excuses for why I was not the best I could be at my sport.

I stepped on the plane back to Ireland with fire in my belly and a plan of action. I spent the next five weeks reading every resource I could get my hands on. I read all about successful sportspeople from every field. The message was the same from every one of them. They didn't do just one thing and they didn't do it alone. Each one of them had a team. They didn't just take advice from a coach: they listened to nutritionists, physiotherapists, psychologists, agents and trusted friends. Okay, so I was only a small fish in Irish athletics. I wasn't even a blip on the radar in international competition. But I knew I could find a way to be as good as I could be and see where that would take me.

I started looking for the best people to help me with different areas of my life. I had no financing to do this, so I worked a telesales job for five hours every day and I spent the rest of every day organising myself, making plans and learning at every opportunity. It was Team Derval: Operation World Domination.

One of the most important people I encountered was a nutritionist by the name of Andrea Cullen. She forever changed my views on health and my approach to food. Andrea is someone that I have huge respect and admiration for. After just one hour in Andrea's company, I changed the way I thought about food. The best thing about working with Andrea was that I didn't end up with an obsessive list of forbidden foods. I actually developed a love of eating healthier foods. Along with receiving expert nutrition advice from Andrea, I was fortunate enough to start working with husband-and-wife coaching team Sean and Terrie Cahill. They left no stone unturned and their approach to performance included every aspect. They turned my world domination plan into medals.

Winter 2004 marked the start of my journey towards being a healthier person. There were some big changes for me. I had slipped into the college way of life of eating processed, cheap canteen food. That habit had to be replaced. I started cooking more and more. I changed how I snacked on foods and I made an effort to prioritise rest and to sleep in a much more regular pattern. I looked at all the aspects of my overall health and saw how they related to my performance. In simple terms: I decided that the healthier I was, the faster I would run.

In March 2006 I stood on the line for the World Indoor Championships and it took me 7.84 seconds to become World Champion. I finally became the athlete I wanted to be.

My journey started out with eating healthy and tasty food. Then this grew into a passion for cooking my own healthy and tasty food. I began experimenting more and more in the kitchen. I competed in my third Olympics in London 2012 and, after the huge build-up and all the pressures that come with an event of that magnitude, I needed a break. I decided to sign up to cookery school and it was one of the best decisions I have ever made. I learned loads and I even ran my fastest time in seven years a couple of months after cookery school!

You don't have to be an elite athlete to care about what goes into your body. Each one of us can spend a bit of time and effort on the health of our bodies and minds. Even if you don't know where to start, just start somewhere. Your health is a priceless asset.

My main fitness tip is just to get up and get out. Getting started is the hardest part of being fit – but if you put your runners on and leave the house, you will always get something done and you will always feel better afterwards. My main health tip is to be aware of what you are eating. Start reading the labels on the food you are buying – it will really open your eyes.

If I've learned one thing in recent years, it's that running fast isn't just about turning up and doing the work in the gym and on the track. It's about what you do with the other twenty hours of the day. My approach to food? It should be tasty and nutritious. My philosophy? Sleep well, eat well and live well.

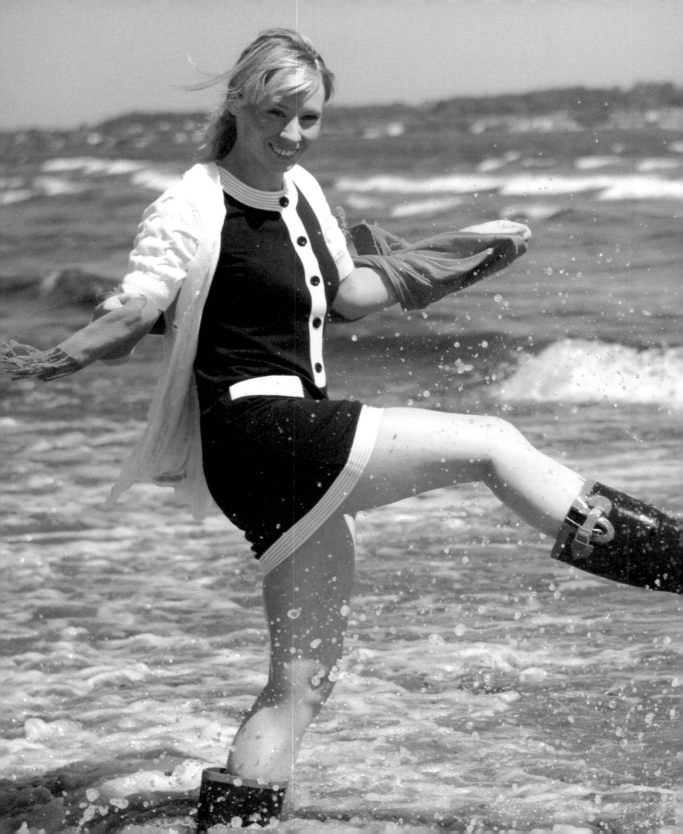

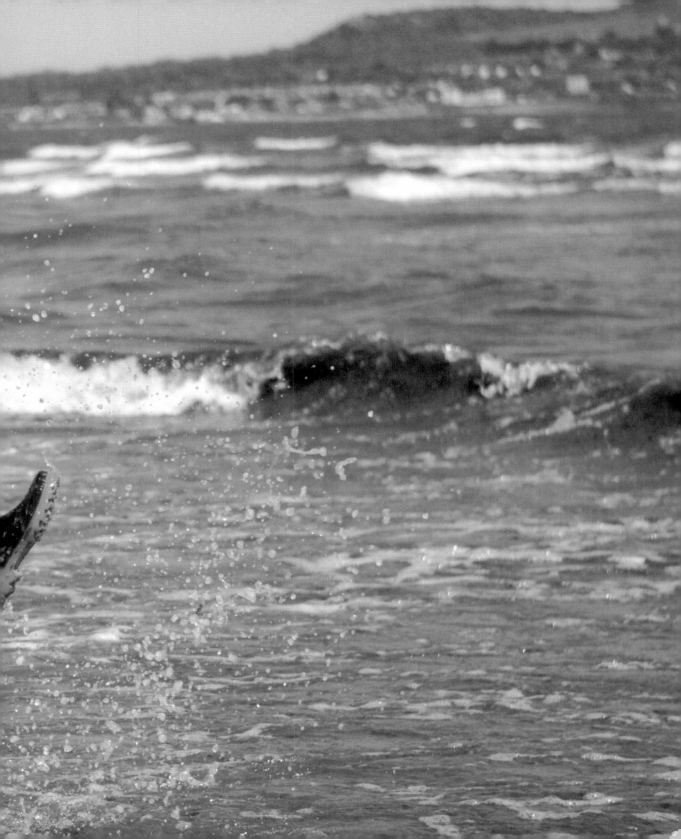

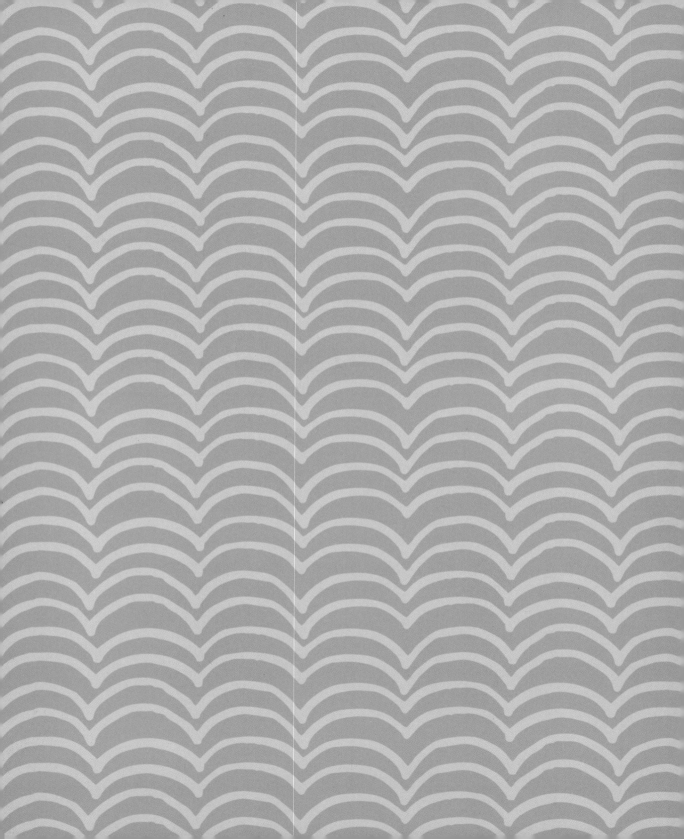

THE FOOD SHOP

If you want to be healthy, you need to fill your cupboards with good ingredients. This means doing efficient and healthy food shops. More times than I can remember, people have come up to me in a supermarket and asked me if they can look in my trolley. Actually, some people don't come up and ask: they just stare in my trolley and act like I can't see them… It sounds completely crazy, but I swear this has happened to me loads of times! At first I used to think it was very odd but now I think it's quite funny and nice that people are interested in the food I'm buying. In honour of the people who find other people's shopping trolleys so interesting, here is a little insight into a standard shopping trolley of mine.

DAIRY: • Full-fat milk • Greek yoghurt • Feta cheese • Goat's cheese

VEGETABLES: • Onions • Garlic • Chilli • Whatever else is in season

FRUIT: • Apples • Bananas • Whatever else is in season

EGGS: • Free-range large eggs

FROZEN: • Vegetables • Fruit

MEAT: • Chicken • Beef • Turkey

FISH: • Whatever is in season

COFFEE & TEA

I love coffee but I try to keep it to one cup a day. I love it either first thing in the morning before training or in the afternoon after my session.

My opinion on coffee is that you don't need a fancy coffee machine: you just need a good grinder, a French press and quality beans. There are loads of great Irish companies producing fab coffee blends. Some of my favourites are 3FE, Java Republic, Badger & Dodo and Red Rooster Coffee.

On the running circuit, almost every athlete drinks coffee. We spend so much time waiting around hotels or airports that a good cup of coffee is always a nice way to pass the time. Coffee and racing go hand in hand, really. No matter how heated and tense the races get, it's always nice to sit down for a cup of coffee after a race with my competitors.

Tea is my other drink. I drink either Barry's Tea or good-quality peppermint tea. If I'm feeling very nervous on the day of a race, I drink peppermint tea: it settles my stomach. Whenever I drink tea at home, it's Barry's.

TIPS FOR THE GROCERY SHOP

1.
Always bring a list. It's ok to veer off the list but at least you won't go home without essential ingredients.

2.
If you can take the time, go to more than just one place. I love going to the butcher, the fruit and vegetable shop and the supermarket.

3.
Avoid the aisle that is full of biscuits, chocolate and sweets. You don't need the temptation.

4.
Look for ingredients lists that are short. The more items that appear on the list, the worse the food product is for you. Products with long lists of ingredients tend to have loads of sugars and additives.

5.
Buy fruit and vegetables in season and locally, where possible. They will be cheaper and they won't have travelled thousands of miles to get to you.

6.
Don't go food shopping when you are hungry, unless you want to make way more impulse purchases than you should.

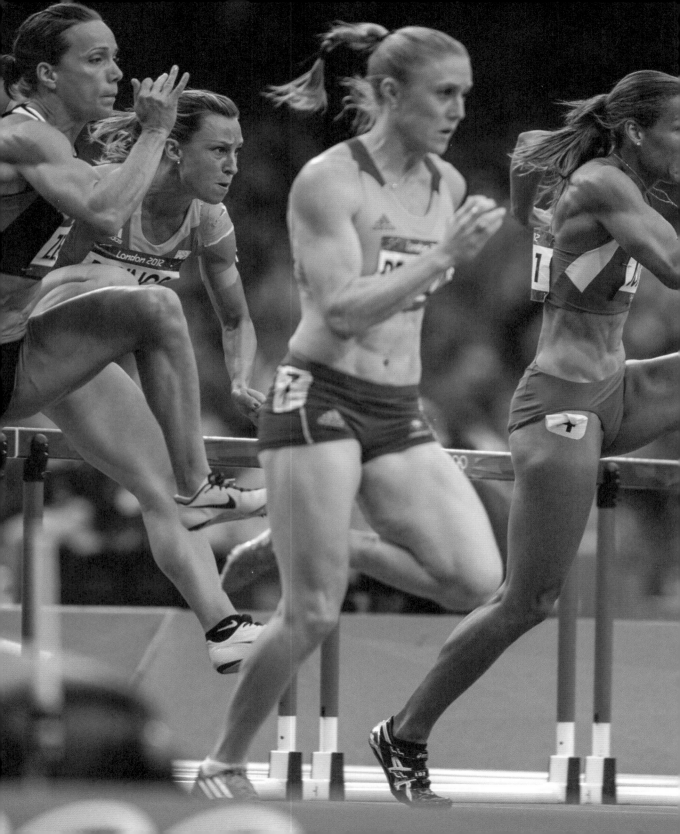

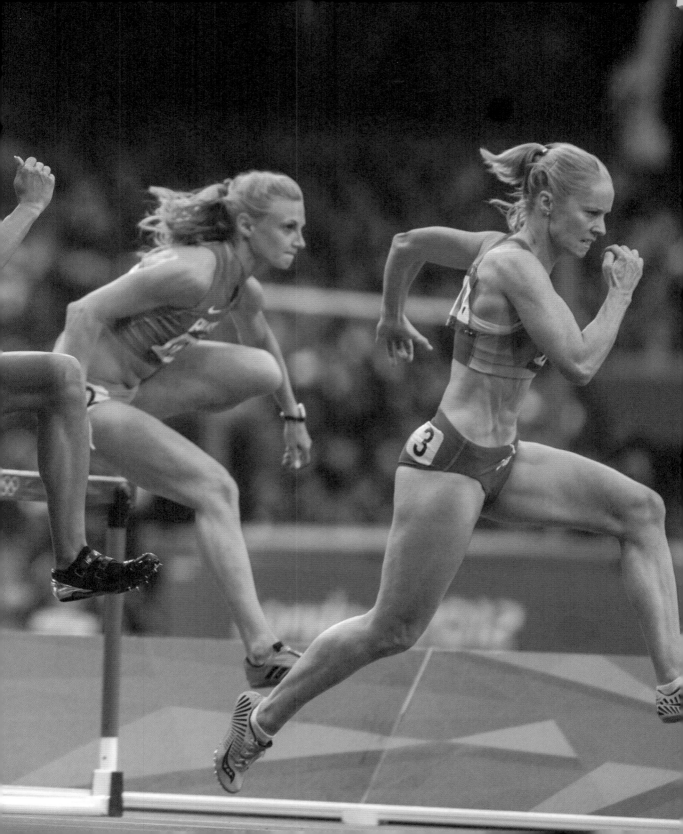

TIPS FOR THE HEALTH FOOD SHOP

I hate recipes that have ingredients that I'll most likely never have in my cupboard or have to spend half a day searching for. In the hope of avoiding Recipe Rage from any readers, I'm making this list of ingredients that you should pick up in the health food shop. These ingredients might be difficult to find in the grocery shop, but if you go to the health food shop once a month and pick up a good supply of these few ingredients, it should be enough to keep you going.

Another pet peeve of mine is a recipe that has so many unusual ingredients that it costs a fortune to make! Some of my recipes include unusual ingredients but, in my defence, if you buy these few items they will last you ages. A good example is my Happy, Healthy Bread (p.135). If you buy a packet of everything on the ingredients list, you will have enough in your cupboards to make Happy, Healthy Bread many times over.

Remember that shopping in the health food shop is similar to shopping anywhere else in the sense that prices can vary greatly. So shop around, be smart and stock up on any offers. A well-stocked cupboard is half the battle when it comes to cooking and eating well.

COCONUT OIL

This is a fairly recent discovery in the health world but it's popping up in loads of recipes. I use it regularly but not exclusively: I like to use olive oil too. Coconut oil is thought to have loads of health benefits from metabolism to immune system. I try to buy the extra-virgin, unrefined version. It can be a little expensive and it is worth buying in bulk if it is on offer. Store it in a cool dry place.

AGAVE SYRUP

I use agave syrup as a natural sweetener. It's similar to honey but research suggests that it has a lower glycemic index, which means that it shouldn't cause a sharp rise or fall in blood sugar levels. This sounds like a win-win to me. Remember that it is still a sweetener, so don't go mad with it!

QUINOA

This is used in a lot of my recipes. It is often found in the supermarket and it is definitely in every health food shop. It is a plant-based, complete protein and is high in fibre. It's a great addition to meals and to life in general. A bit of a superstar food, really.

PROTEIN POWDER

I buy this in the health food shop or online. See p.52 for my take on supplements. Many of the recipes in this book contain vanilla, banana or chocolate flavoured protein powders.

GRAM FLOUR

This is chickpea flour. Put simply: it is ground-up chickpeas. I like to use it instead of wheat flour in some recipes. It will also thicken soups. It contains no gluten, which is handy if you are trying to reduce your gluten intake or are on a gluten-free diet.

COCONUT FLOUR

I love coconut; this is what led me to coconut flour. I use it a little in baking but it is difficult to work with: recipes can turn out dry with coconut flour. On the positive side, it is gluten-free. So experiment with your recipes: try using coconut flour and adding a little extra liquid in your baking.

PSYLLIUM HUSK

This is a key ingredient in my Happy, Healthy Bread. Buy one bag and it will last you for ages.

SAMBUCOL

This little potion combats flu and cold symptoms. It's made out of elderberry extract and is far better than any other product I've ever taken when I've been sick. I always keep a bottle in the house. It's a cold remedy so it doesn't appear in any of my recipes – but I still think you should buy it.

HEALTHY ALTERNATIVES

I think life is too short to exclude the things I love. Rather than having a list of meals that are off-limits because they contain certain ingredients, I find ways to adapt my meals to incorporate healthier alternatives. Most of the time, it works brilliantly and it's a guilt-free way of eating any meal I want.

I love to take a recipe and make substitutions for any of the ingredients that could do with a healthier alternative. So, rather than using white flour and white sugar, I'll try the recipe with spelt flour and agave syrup. Many of the recipes in this book came about because I was experimenting in this way. If you want to give it a go yourself, here's a handy chart to get you started.

ORIGINAL	ALTERNATIVE
White sugar	Agave syrup
Cooking oil	Coconut oil
Cream	Natural yoghurt
Mayonnaise	Greek yoghurt
White flour	Gram, coconut or spelt flour
White rice	Brown rice or quinoa
White pasta	Wholewheat pasta
White bread	Brown bread or rye bread

DERVAL'S COOKING TIPS & TRICKS

When you are SHOPPING FOR LEEKS, the best ones to buy are the fat ones that have loads of white.

BASIL should be chopped once only: otherwise it will turn black.

It is no harm to add a little SALT to your food as you are cooking. This helps to bring out the flavour and it means that you don't have to add salt at the end of cooking.

After MAKING FRESH STOCK, wait for it to cool. Freeze it in an ice-cube tray and use it straight from the freezer as needed.

When using FRESH HERBS, it is important to distinguish whether they are hard or soft herbs. Hard herbs (e.g. tarragon, rosemary and thyme) may be added in at the start of the cooking process, since these herbs will hold their flavour. Soft herbs (e.g. basil, mint, dill, parsley, coriander and chives) must be added in as a finishing herb, otherwise they will lose their flavour.

MAKING SOUP does not need to be tedious. Soup can cook quickly if you cut all the vegetables into small pieces. Do spend time on the first stage of the soup, though: sweating onion or celery for about 10 minutes is always time well spent.

Keep lots of containers for storing LEFTOVERS.

If you regularly cook with FRESH GARLIC but do not want to keep preparing it fresh each time, finely chop a quantity that is large enough for a few days of cooking. Cover the chopped garlic in olive oil, store it in the fridge and use as needed.

MEAT cooks better when it is at room temperature, so take it out of the fridge at least 30 minutes before you use it.

When PAN-FRYING, add a dash of water if the pan starts to look dry.

POTATO and GRAM FLOUR are great thickeners for soup (and it is nicer than using wheat flour).

Make your own SALAD DRESSINGS –
see p.132 for some of my recipes.

Add SPICES at the beginning of cooking to bring out their flavours.

POACHING EGGS takes a bit of practice. For best results, use a big pot, the freshest eggs and a good glug of vinegar in the water.

Store HERBS in a cool dark place – keep them away from the cooker.

The FREEZER is a great resource. Whenever you can, cook in batches and freeze for later.

FOOD & FITNESS DIARY

Over the years I have completed loads of Food & Fitness Diaries for my coaching team. It's a really good exercise to do because it lays out everything in front of you and makes you accountable for the choices you have made. Sometimes our perception of what we are doing in terms of food and exercise is vastly different from the reality. The whole point of a Food & Fitness Diary is truth-telling. Be honest: no leaving out that sneaky glass of wine or packet of crisps!

Below is one of my real-life Food & Fitness Diaries over the course of one week. This training schedule was off-season when I was doing lots of fitness work. It's worth noting that I have a pretty heavy exercise routine (being an athlete is my job, after all) so my food intake is high! However, you could use this template as a way to start tracking your own food and exercise habits so that you can make a plan that's right for your life.

BREAKFAST	Summer Oats
	Cup of coffee
TRAINING SESSION	Weights

Warm-up
Mobility exercises: 15kg weights bar;
3 sets of 8 lifts; Overhead Squat, Back Squat
and Good Morning Stretching

Session
Snatch: 3 sets of 5 lifts at 30kg, 35kg and 40kg
3 sets of lifts at 45kg, 47.5kg and 50kg
Front Squat: 4 sets of 10 lifts at 45kg, 50kg
and 55kg
Row: 3 sets of 10 reps at 15kg
Medicine Ball: Throws at the wall, 3 sets of 10

Warm down
Stretching and core exercises

LOCKER-ROOM SNACK	Peter's Frozen Protein Bar
LUNCH	Spicy Chicken Pitta
AFTERNOON SNACK	Sliced apple with almond butter
	Sprinter Spritzer: Vitamin C Boost
DINNER	Steak Salad
NIGHT-TIME SNACK	A few squares of dark chocolate

MONDAY

BREAKFAST	Power Pancake
TRAINING SESSION	Running

Warm-up

10-minute jog,
stretching and drills over 30m

Session

150m x 3 runs, 120m x 3 runs
and 90m x 3 runs: all at 85% effort

Warm down

Hurdle drills, 10-minute jog
and 10 minutes core

LOCKER-ROOM SNACK	Super Snacks
LUNCH	Enchiladas
	Sprinter Spritzer: Lemony Goodness
AFTERNOON SNACK	Quick Choccie Chip Cookies
DINNER	Jogger's Beef Stew
NIGHT-TIME SNACK	Sweet & Sticky Pecans
	Peppermint tea

BREAKFAST	Stopwatch Brown Bread with mashed avocado and boiled egg
	Cup of coffee
TRAINING SESSION	Weights

Warm-up

Mobility exercises: 15kg weights bar; 3 sets of 8 lifts;
Overhead Squat, Back Squat and Good Morning Stretching

Session

Power clean: 4 sets of 5 lifts at 45kg, 50kg, 55kg and 60kg
3 sets of 3 lifts at 65kg, 67.5kg and 70kg

Back Squat: 4 sets of 10 lifts at 50kg, 60kg, 70kg and 75kg

Chin-ups: 4 sets of 6

Swiss Ball: Hamstring roll-outs, 4 sets of 10

Warm down

Core exercises: 4 sets of 10

LOCKER-ROOM SNACK	Banana Protein Smoothie: Almond & Vanilla
LUNCH	Fiery Spaghetti
AFTERNOON SNACK	Pitta Chips with dips
DINNER	Grilled Salmon with Celeriac Spinach Mash
NIGHT-TIME SNACK	Happy, Healthy Bread with butter

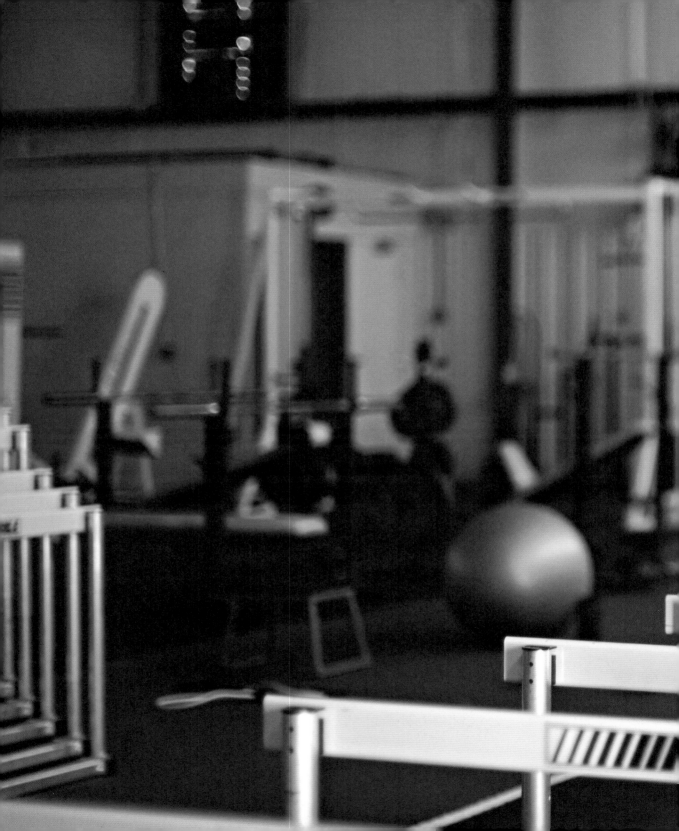

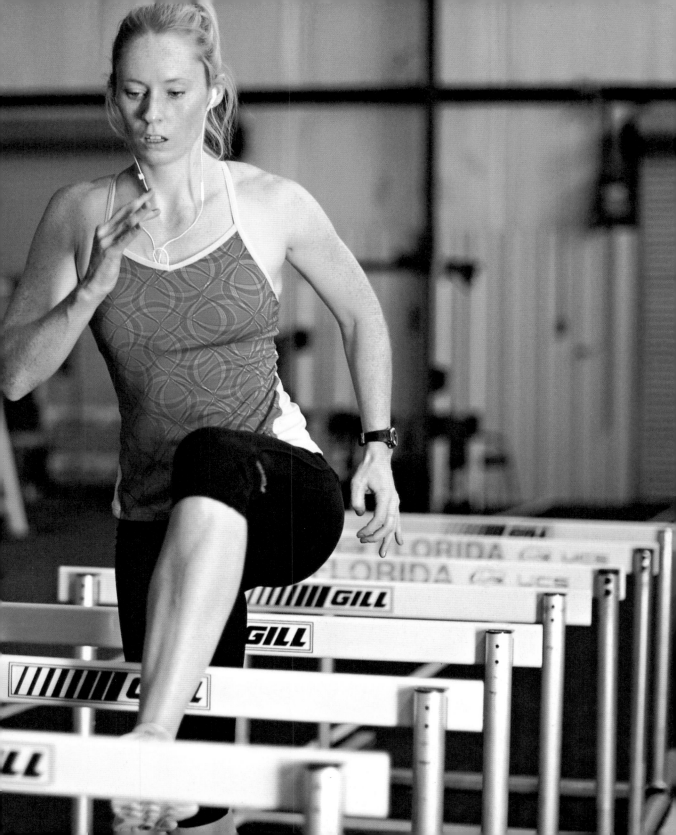

BREAKFAST	Granola with Greek yoghurt and banana
	Boiled egg
TRAINING SESSION:	Running
	Warm-up
	10-minute jog, stretching and drills over 30m
	Session
	200m x 2 runs, 180m x 1 run, 160m x 2 runs and
	120m x 1 run: all at 75% effort
	Hurdles drills while jogging
	Warm down
	Hurdle drills, 10-minute jog and 10 minutes core
LOCKER-ROOM SNACK	Great Balls of Power
LUNCH	Chicken & Vegetable Soup
	Stopwatch Brown Bread
AFTERNOON SNACK	Dark Chocolate & Orange Zest Brownie
DINNER	Stuffed Peppers
NIGHT-TIME SNACK	Double Decker bar (all work and no play…)
	Cup of tea

BREAKFAST	Breakfast Beans
	Stopwatch Brown Bread
	Cup of coffee
TRAINING SESSION	Recovery day
SNACK	Sweet & Sticky Pecans
LUNCH	Chicken Salad with Beetroot, Carrot & Quinoa
AFTERNOON SNACK	Super Snacks
	Cup of tea
DINNER	Dinner out!
	Starter: crab salad. Mains: steak with potatoes.
	Dessert: ice cream to share
NIGHT-TIME SNACK	That's enough now: stuffed from eating out

BREAKFAST	Baked Avocado, Eggs & Basil
	Cup of coffee
TRAINING SESSION:	Running and speed session

Warm-up
10-minute jog, stretching and drills over 30m, hurdle drills

Session
80m x 2 runs, 60m x 3 runs and 40m x 3 runs
Hurdle jogging drills

Warm down
10-minute jog and range of movement exercises

LOCKER-ROOM SNACK	Brunch out!
	Scrambled eggs, brown bread and a glass of fresh juice
LUNCH	[Had brunch]
AFTERNOON SNACK	Go Bananas!
DINNER	Baked Hake & Smashed Spuds
NIGHT-TIME SNACK	A few squares of dark chocolate
	Peppermint tea

BREAKFAST	Summer Oats
TRAINING SESSION:	Hill running

Warm-up
15-minute jog and stretching

Session
Hill: 200m, 180m, 150m x 3 runs x 3 sets

Warm down
10-minute gentle jog and 5 minutes core

LOCKER-ROOM SNACK	Great Balls of Power
LUNCH	Creamy Tomato & Cannellini Bean Soup
AFTERNOON SNACK	Lemon Drizzle & Poppy Seed Square
	Cup of tea
DINNER	Roast Chicken, Sweet Potato Mash, Red Cabbage & Apple
NIGHT-TIME SNACK	Greek yoghurt sprinkled with Granola

HEALTHY HABITS CALENDAR

If you get into the habit of doing things in a healthy way, you can't go wrong: the habit seems to take over. It's a good idea to work on one habit at a time, until you see real change. Here are twelve new habits to try: one for each month of the year.

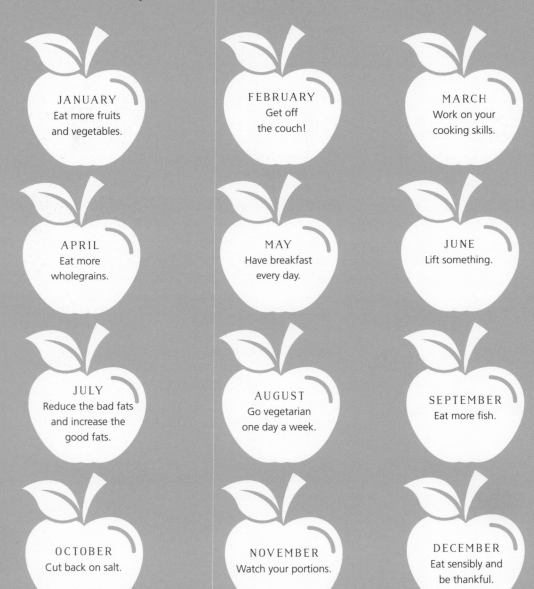

JANUARY
Eat more fruits
and vegetables.

FEBRUARY
Get off
the couch!

MARCH
Work on your
cooking skills.

APRIL
Eat more
wholegrains.

MAY
Have breakfast
every day.

JUNE
Lift something.

JULY
Reduce the bad fats
and increase the
good fats.

AUGUST
Go vegetarian
one day a week.

SEPTEMBER
Eat more fish.

OCTOBER
Cut back on salt.

NOVEMBER
Watch your portions.

DECEMBER
Eat sensibly and
be thankful.

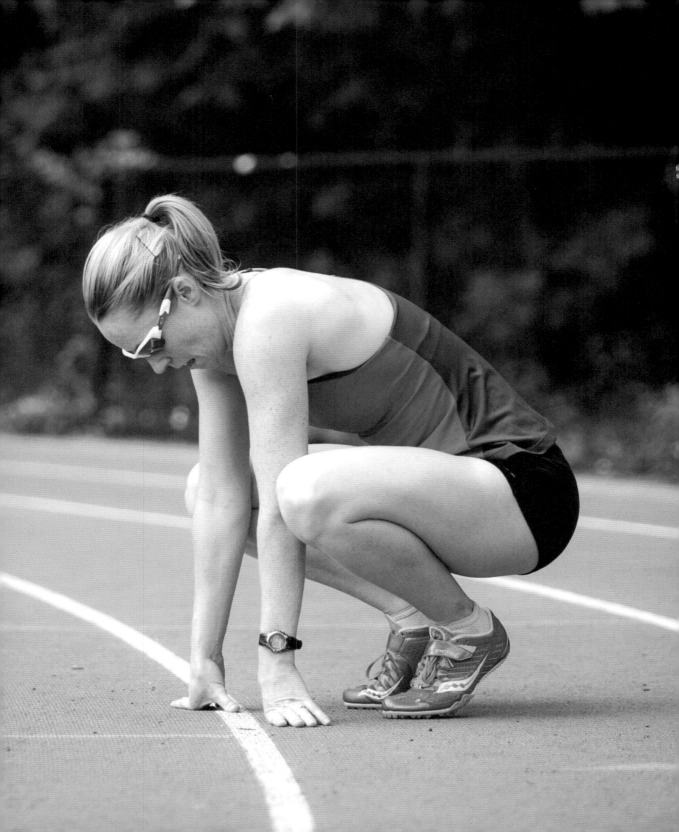

BREAKFAST

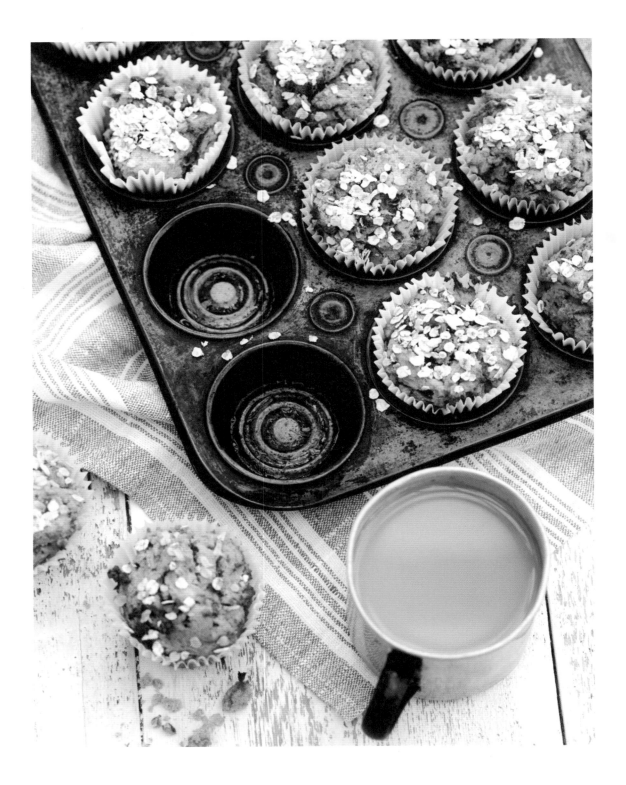

APPLE & CARROT MUFFINS

These make a brilliant snack with a cup of tea. They're warm and hearty and they smell like Christmas because of the cinnamon, nutmeg and cloves. Store these muffins in an airtight container: they'll keep at room temperature for several days or in the fridge for about a week.

GET THE MUFFIN - NOT THE MUFFIN TOP!

MAKES 8 LARGE MUFFINS

70g wholemeal flour
40g plain flour
20g chopped walnuts
1 tsp ground cinnamon
1 tsp baking powder
½ tsp ground nutmeg
¼ tsp salt (optional)
¼ tsp ground cloves (optional)
1 eating apple (such as Pink Lady),
   peeled, cored and grated
1 large carrot, peeled and grated
4 large eggs
4 dates, pitted and finely chopped
4 tbsp natural yoghurt
4 tbsp coconut oil
1 tbsp agave syrup
1 tsp vanilla extract

Preheat the oven to 180°C/350°F/gas 4. Line a muffin tin with 8 deep paper cases.

Mix the flours, walnuts, cinnamon, baking powder, nutmeg, salt and cloves in a small bowl and set aside.

Place the apple and carrot in a large mixing bowl and blot them with kitchen paper to remove excess moisture. Add the eggs, dates, yoghurt, coconut oil, agave syrup and vanilla extract and stir well. Pour the dry ingredients into the wet ingredients and mix until just combined.

Use a spoon to divide the batter evenly among the paper cases, so that they are almost full. Bake for 25 minutes until the muffins are golden brown and a skewer inserted comes out clean. Carefully remove the muffins from the tin and allow to cool on a wire rack.

POWER PANCAKE

Traditional pancakes are not a food I'd reach for because of their nutritional value, so I went in search of a healthy alternative. This Power Pancake is high in protein, which is perfect for a nutritional breakfast. A Power Pancake is also a pre-weight-training favourite for me. My weights coach, Martina McCarthy, loves these.

○ ○

SERVES 1

½ banana, peeled and mashed
20g porridge oats
1 scoop of vanilla protein powder
1 egg white
1 tbsp milk
¼ tsp cinnamon
1 tsp coconut oil
2 tbsp Granola (p.24), to serve
1 tbsp Greek yoghurt, to serve
fresh berries, to serve

Stir the banana, oats, vanilla protein powder, egg white, milk and cinnamon in a small bowl to make a paste.

Heat a 20cm (8 inch) non-stick pan until very hot, then add the coconut oil. Once the coconut oil has melted, pour in the pancake batter. Quickly swirl the pan to spread the batter and use a spatula to loosen the edge of the pancake away from the pan. Cook for 2 minutes. Use a spatula to lift the edge of the pancake to see if it's cooked underneath. As soon as it's golden, flip it over and cook for 2 minutes on the other side. Slide the cooked pancake onto a warmed serving plate and top with the Granola, Greek yoghurt and berries.

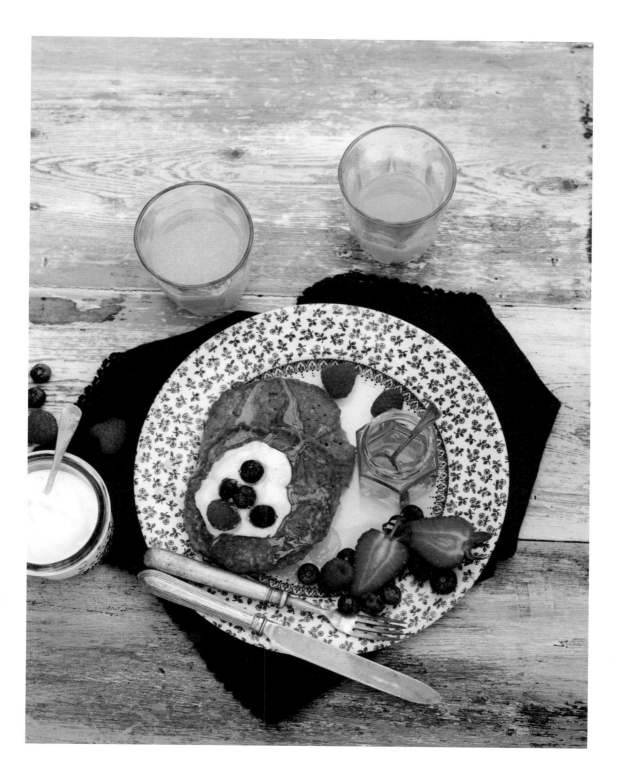

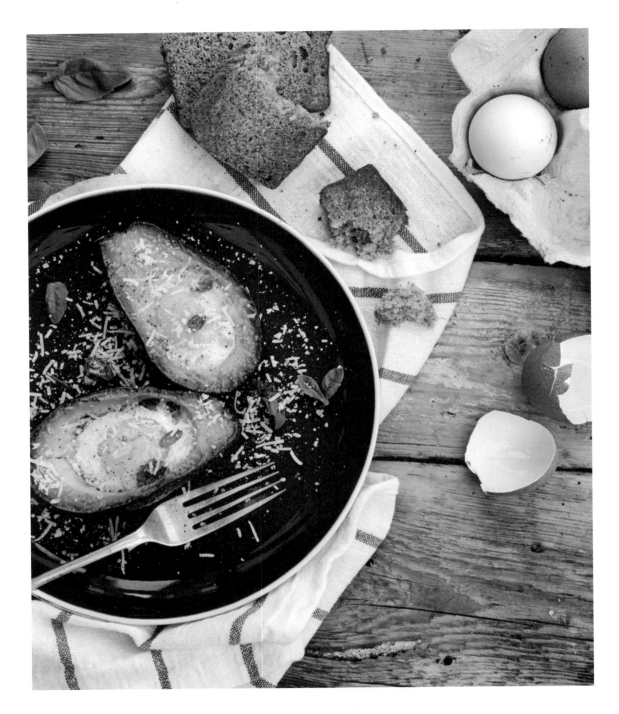

EXPECT CHALLENGES - AND EAT THEM FOR BREAKFAST!

BAKED AVOCADO, EGGS & BASIL

This is a lovely weekend breakfast or brunch recipe. It takes a little time, with the eggs being baked in the oven. On Saturday mornings, I don't have to be out training quite as early as I do on other mornings. So this recipe is perfect for those times when I have the extra hour to shuffle around the kitchen and make something nice.

○ ○

SERVES 2

1 avocado
salt and pepper
a few basil leaves, chopped
2 eggs
grated Parmesan, to garnish
Stopwatch Brown Bread
(p.134), to serve

Preheat the oven to 180°C/350°F/gas 4.

Cut the avocado in half and remove the stone. Use a teaspoon to scoop out some of the flesh from each avocado half, creating a hollow large enough to hold a cracked egg. Chop the scooped-out avocado flesh and set aside.

Season the avocado halves and sprinkle an equal amount of chopped basil over each one, reserving some basil as a garnish. Crack one egg into each avocado half.

Place the filled avocado halves on a baking tray, being careful not to spill the eggs. Bake for 20 minutes.

Arrange the baked avocado halves on serving plates alongside the chopped avocado. Garnish with the basil and Parmesan and serve with Stopwatch Brown Bread.

> I'M NOT A BIG CEREAL PERSON. I HAVE NEVER LOVED BREAKFAST CEREAL THE WAY A LOT OF PEOPLE DO. BUT I DO LOVE PORRIDGE OATS AND THEY ARE GOOD ALL YEAR ROUND.

SUMMER OATS

These oats are perfect for the summer months because you don't have to cook them. You just mix everything together and the recipe takes care of itself overnight in the fridge. The next morning you can add whatever topping you like.

SERVES 1

50g porridge oats
120ml Greek yogurt
120ml milk or rice milk
1 tsp chia seeds
½ tsp vanilla extract

Combine all of the ingredients in a large bowl. Transfer the mixture to a serving bowl, cover and leave to soak overnight in the fridge.

Next morning, add the topping of your choice and serve.

WINTER OATS

When winter comes around, I need my oats. I would never get through hard winter training without a bowl of hot porridge in the mornings. Winter oats always make me think of wild Irish weather and running up hills in Dalgan Park on a Sunday morning.

SERVES 1

50g porridge oats
120ml milk
120ml water
1 tbsp wheat germ

Combine the oats, milk and water in a small pan over a medium heat. Cook gently, stirring occasionally, until the porridge is soft and creamy. Pour the porridge into a serving bowl, sprinkle over the wheat germ and serve.

TOPPINGS

These toppings are great with Summer Oats and Winter Oats:

- Chopped banana, crushed pecans and a drizzle of agave syrup • Blueberries and sliced strawberries
- Grated apple and crushed raw cashews • Chopped medjool dates and a drizzle of agave.

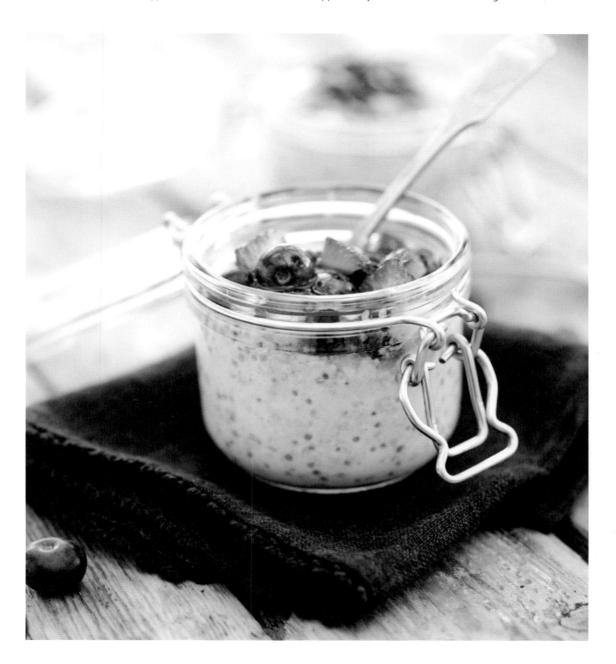

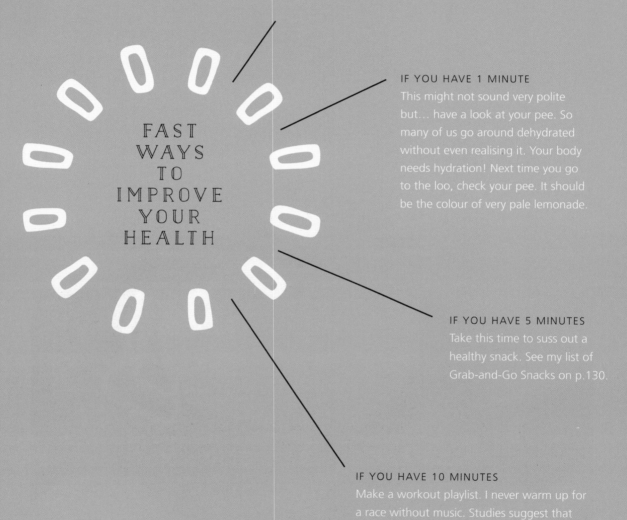

IF YOU HAVE 30 SECONDS
Grab a handful of nuts: they are packed with protein, fibre and essential fats. I keep nuts in my bag and spend half my life digging them out and munching on them.

FAST WAYS TO IMPROVE YOUR HEALTH

IF YOU HAVE 1 MINUTE
This might not sound very polite but… have a look at your pee. So many of us go around dehydrated without even realising it. Your body needs hydration! Next time you go to the loo, check your pee. It should be the colour of very pale lemonade.

IF YOU HAVE 5 MINUTES
Take this time to suss out a healthy snack. See my list of Grab-and-Go Snacks on p.130.

IF YOU HAVE 10 MINUTES
Make a workout playlist. I never warm up for a race without music. Studies suggest that listening to music on the move cuts the perceived effort. I'm pretty sure Jay-Z is responsible for many of my Irish records.

DON'T SIT - GET FIT

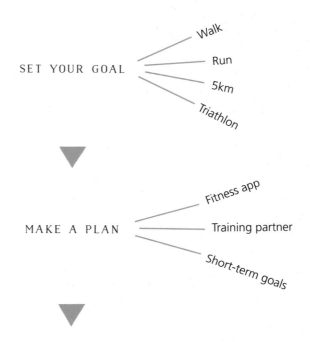

SET YOUR GOAL
- Walk
- Run
- 5km
- Triathlon

MAKE A PLAN
- Fitness app
- Training partner
- Short-term goals

ACHIEVE YOUR GOAL —— Yippee!

REPEAT

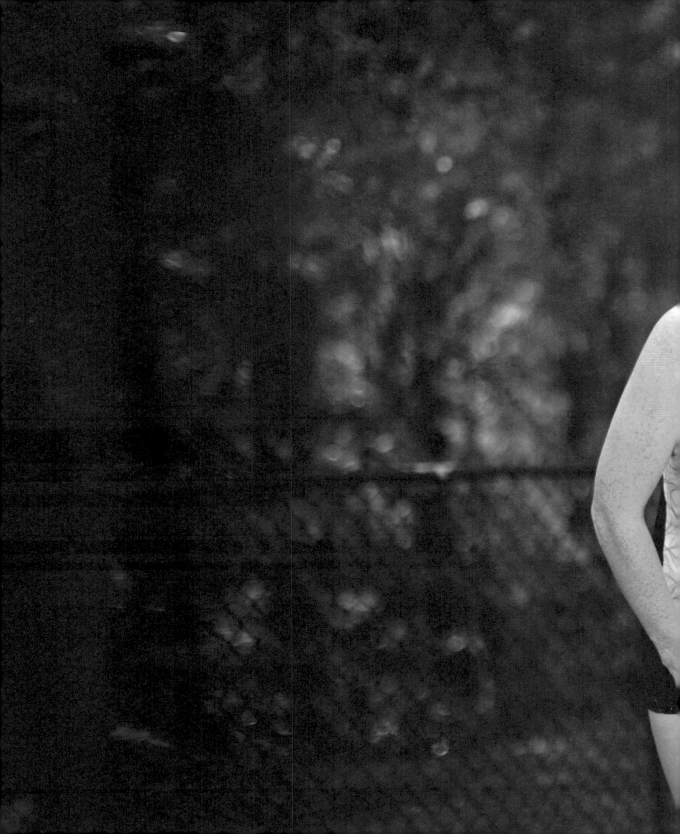

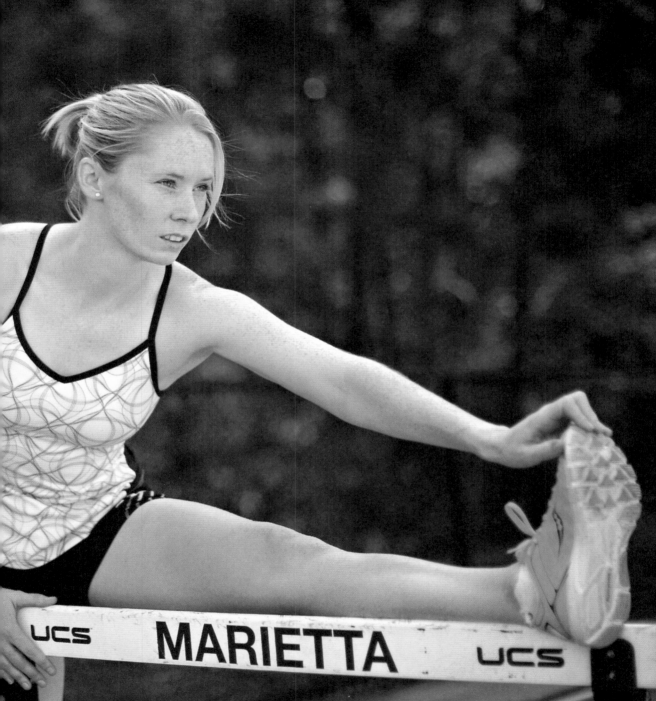

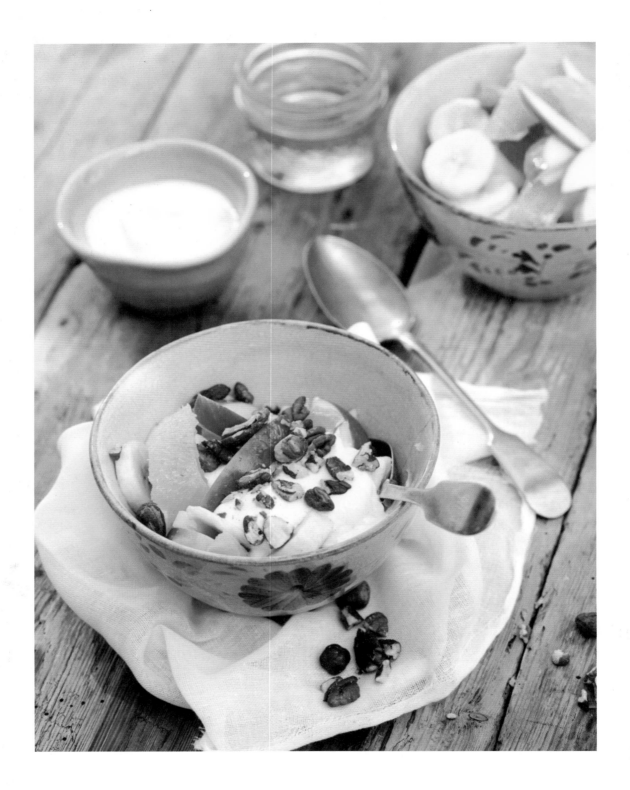

FRUIT BOWL

It goes without saying that fruit is the smart choice when it comes to snacking – and a little bit of extra effort really pays off. I often have this for breakfast: it's a handy way to use up leftover fruit and it goes really well with a cup of coffee too.

If I want to pack in a little protein, I'll have this with a boiled egg on the side.

SERVES 1

3 different pieces of fruit, such as
banana, apple and plum
2–3 tbsp Greek yoghurt or another
yoghurt of your choice
2 tbsp mixed nuts
1 tsp agave syrup or honey

Prepare your chosen fruits into bite-sized pieces and place them in a serving bowl. Pour in the yoghurt, sprinkle over the nuts, drizzle over the agave syrup and serve.

SCRAMBLED EGGS & SPINACH

I like to eat some protein in the mornings, so scrambled eggs are a great start to my day. They go really well with a slice of brown or nutty bread. Spinach adds lovely flavour here and it's a food that's packed full of nutrients. It has great anti-inflammatory properties: I reach for it any time I'm recovering from injury.

SERVES 1
2 eggs
3 tbsp milk
a small handful of baby spinach
2 tbsp chopped fresh herbs
salt and pepper

Heat a frying pan over a medium heat. Lightly beat the eggs and milk in a large bowl, add the spinach and herbs and mix well. Tip this mixture into the frying pan. Gently cook the eggs and spinach for 2–3 minutes, stirring occasionally. Then stir in the butter and cook until the eggs are thickened and glossy. Spoon the eggs onto a warmed serving plate, season to taste and serve.

GO BANANAS!

I catch loads of early flights for races, which means that I'm often getting to the airport before the sun has even thought about coming up. Rather than stumble around my kitchen in a sleepy haze looking for something to eat on the morning of a flight, I make this banana recipe the night before and pop it in the fridge so that it's ready to go as soon as I am.

○ ○

SERVES 1

40g jumbo porridge oats

¼ tsp cinnamon

a pinch of salt (optional)

1 banana, peeled and unsliced

2–3 tbsp almond butter or another nut butter of your choice

Mix the oats, cinnamon and salt together and spread out on a plate. Cover the banana with almond butter. Roll the banana in the oat mixture. Place the coated banana in an airtight container and leave it in the fridge overnight. Next morning, grab and go!

RUN LIKE YOU'VE JUST STOLEN SOMETHING!

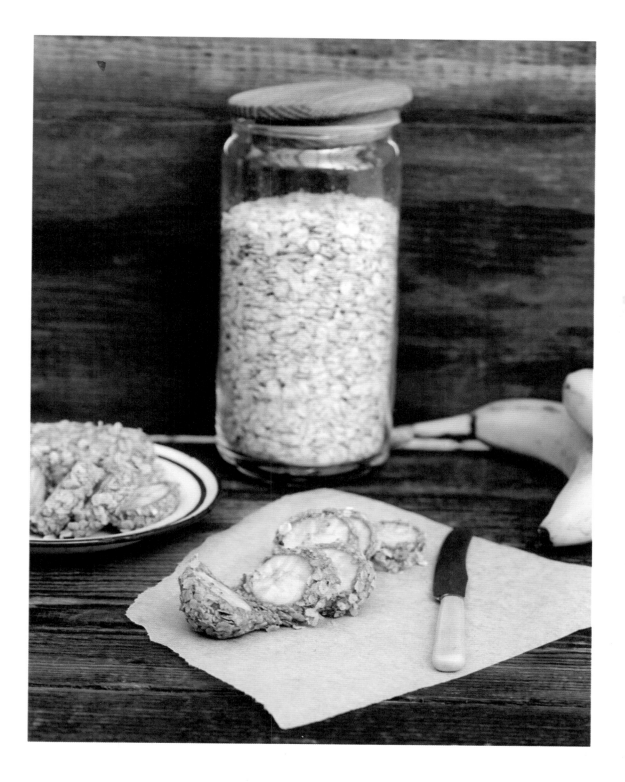

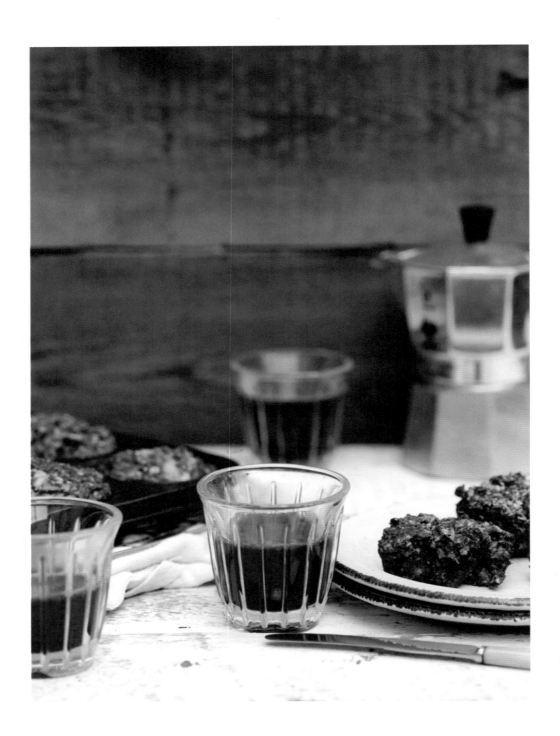

OATY BREAKFAST MUFFINS

I had to teach myself to eat breakfast. I've never liked the idea of sitting down for an hour in the mornings to eat a big meal. I much prefer to grab a coffee and a muffin and get going, so I had to come up with a recipe that would make this a healthy choice.

The best thing about these muffins is that you can do a half-and-half batch, so this recipe makes six Banana Pecan and six Chocolate Coconut in one go. It's like a coffee shop in your kitchen.

MAKES 12 MUFFINS
250g Greek yoghurt
120g jumbo porridge oats
100g agave syrup
70g ground linseed
2 tsp baking powder

For the Banana Pecan:

1 banana, peeled and mashed
50g pecan nuts, roughly chopped

For the Chocolate Coconut:

30g dark chocolate (70% cocoa solids), chopped
30g desiccated coconut

Preheat the oven to 180°C/350°F/gas 4. Line a muffin tin with 12 deep paper cases.

Mix the Greek yoghurt, oats, agave syrup, linseed and baking powder in a large bowl. Then remove half of this mixture to a separate large bowl.

Stir the banana and pecans into the first large bowl, mixing until just combined. Stir the dark chocolate and coconut into the second large bowl, mixing until just combined.

Use a spoon to divide the Banana Pecan batter evenly among 6 of the paper cases, so that they are almost full. Repeat with the Chocolate Coconut batter.

Bake for 15–20 minutes until the muffins are golden and a skewer inserted comes out clean. Carefully remove the muffins from the tin and allow to cool on a wire rack.

BREAKFAST POWER COOKIES

I like to have a really fast on-the-run option in the mornings. No matter how well prepared I am, there are always a few mornings where I don't have time to make breakfast. That's when I turn to a Breakfast Power Cookie.

The cookies have a hearty texture and a little sweetness and they're not just for emergency breakfasts. They are like regular cookies without any of the bad ingredients, so they're a lovely addition to an afternoon cup of tea or coffee (they dunk pretty well too). The cookies keep well in an airtight container for about ten days.

MAKES 15–20 COOKIES

350g rice flour

100g desiccated coconut

100g ground linseed

100g pumpkin seeds

100g sunflower seeds

1 tsp cinnamon

1 tsp salt

50g dark chocolate (70% cocoa solids), chopped

2 eggs

100g agave syrup

200ml coconut oil

1 tsp vanilla extract

Preheat the oven to 180°C/350°F/gas 4. Line two large baking sheets with parchment paper.

Mix the rice flour, coconut, linseed, pumpkin seeds, sunflower seeds, cinnamon, salt and dark chocolate in a large bowl and set aside.

Mix the eggs, agave syrup, coconut oil and vanilla extract in a large bowl. Pour the wet ingredients into the dry ingredients and mix well to form a cookie dough. Roll into balls and place a few centimetres apart on the prepared baking sheets, using your hands to flatten the cookies slightly.

Bake for 15–20 minutes or until golden brown. Allow the cookies to cool slightly on the baking sheets before removing to a wire rack.

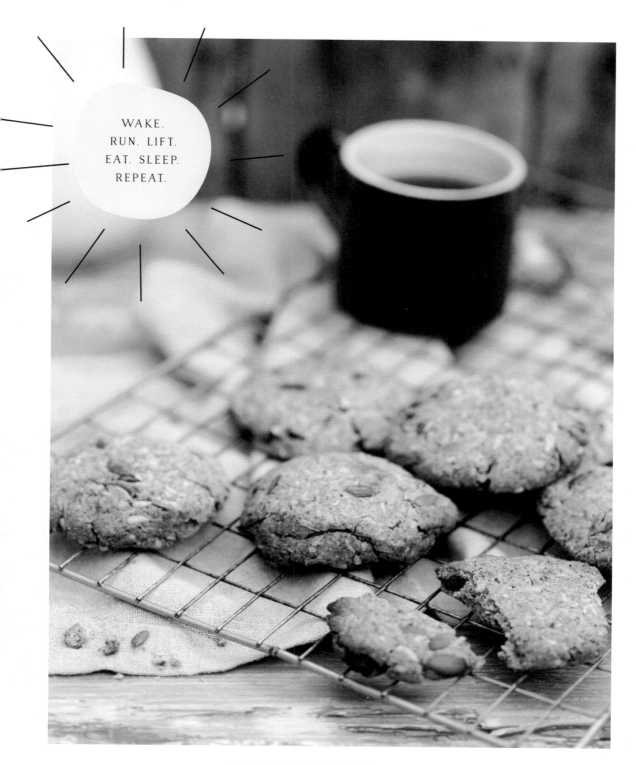

WAKE.
RUN. LIFT.
EAT. SLEEP.
REPEAT.

- THESE COOKIES FREEZE WELL -

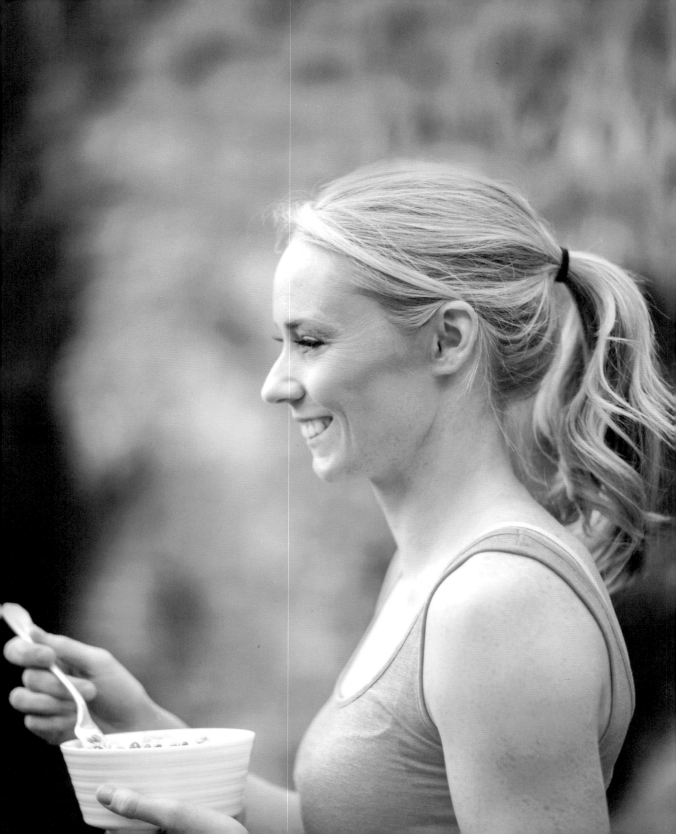

BREAKFAST BEANS

There are two ways to make these beans. The Sprint Method is done on the hob and means you'll have breakfast in 30 minutes. The Marathon Method is prepared the night before and will take 20 minutes in the oven the next morning, giving the beans a lovely crispy finish.

Whichever method you choose, make a big batch: any leftovers can be reheated on the hob for up to a few days afterwards. My grandfather-in-law calls these 'torpedo beans' because they're pretty spicy! If you don't want them too spicy, leave out the chilli.

SERVES 2–3

2 tbsp coconut oil
1 small shallot, finely chopped
1 garlic clove, crushed
1 tbsp smoked paprika
1 tsp chilli flakes (or ½ tsp chopped fresh chilli)
6 thin slices of spicy chorizo, halved (optional)
1 tsp tomato purée
400g tin of chopped tomatoes
400g tin of cannellini, kidney or haricot beans, drained
salt and pepper
Happy, Healthy Bread (p. 135) or crackers, to serve (optional)

Sprint method

Heat the coconut oil in a large pan over a medium heat. Add the shallot and cook for about 10 minutes, until softened. Lower the heat, add the garlic and cook for 1–2 minutes, being careful not to burn it. Add the paprika, chilli flakes and chorizo and cook for 1 minute. Stir in the tomato purée and chopped tomatoes. Simmer, uncovered, for about 20 minutes, stirring occasionally. Add the cannellini beans and simmer for a further 5 minutes. Season to taste. Ladle the beans onto warmed serving plates and serve with Happy, Healthy Bread or crackers.

Marathon method

Combine all of the ingredients in an ovenproof dish and store in the fridge overnight. In the morning, preheat the oven to 180°C/350°F/gas 4. Bake the beans for 20 minutes, until they are piping hot with a crispy top.

GRANOLA

I get frustrated at shop-bought granola and granola recipes that are loaded with butter and sugar. It is totally unnecessary to eat unhealthy granola when healthy granola is so easy to make. You can eat this granola for breakfast, as a snack or as a dessert topping. If I'm going on a long drive, I'll throw a handful of it into a sandwich bag so that I've something nutritious to munch on in the car.

I have made this granola with all sorts of nuts and seeds – it works every time. And once the granola has cooled, you can stir in dried fruits, such as mango, pineapple, raisins or goji berries. This granola will keep in an airtight container for up to two weeks.

MAKES ENOUGH FOR 1 WEEK
100g spelt porridge flakes or jumbo
   porridge oats
50g flaked almonds
50g hazelnuts, crushed
50g pumpkin seeds
50g sunflower seeds
50g walnuts
6 tbsp coconut oil, melted
3 tbsp agave syrup
a pinch of salt

Preheat the oven to 180°/350°F/gas 4. Place all of the ingredients in a large bowl and mix until combined. Tip the granola into an ovenproof dish and bake for 30 minutes, stirring occasionally. Remove from the oven and leave to cool.

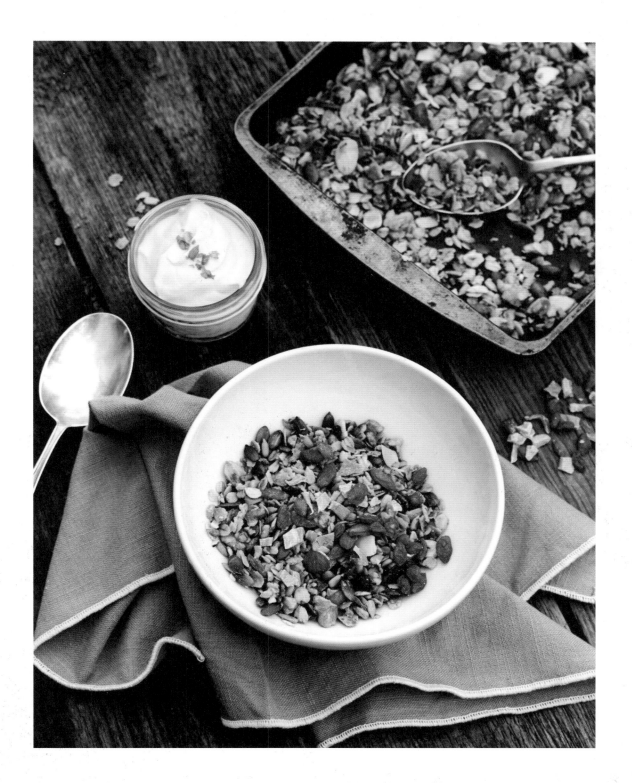

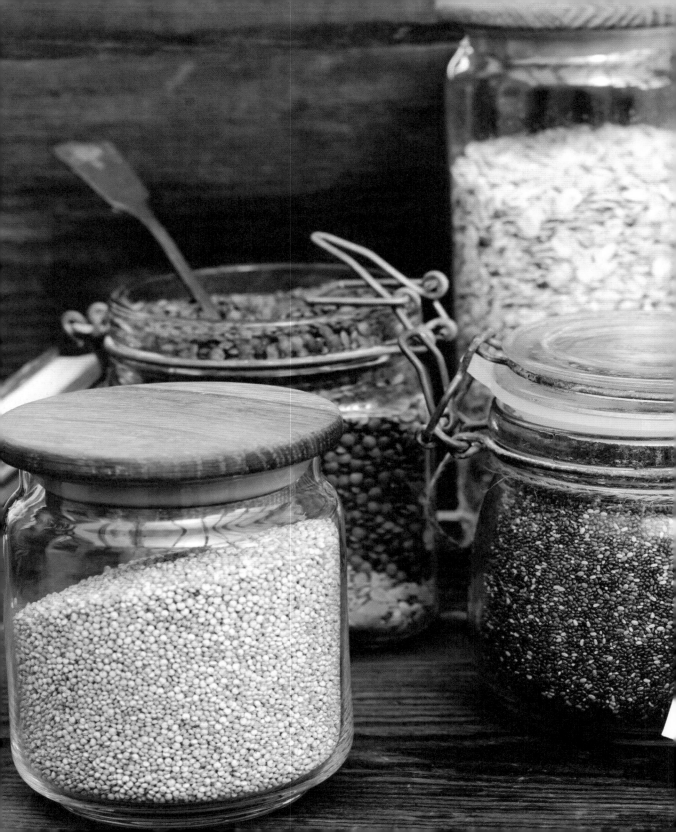

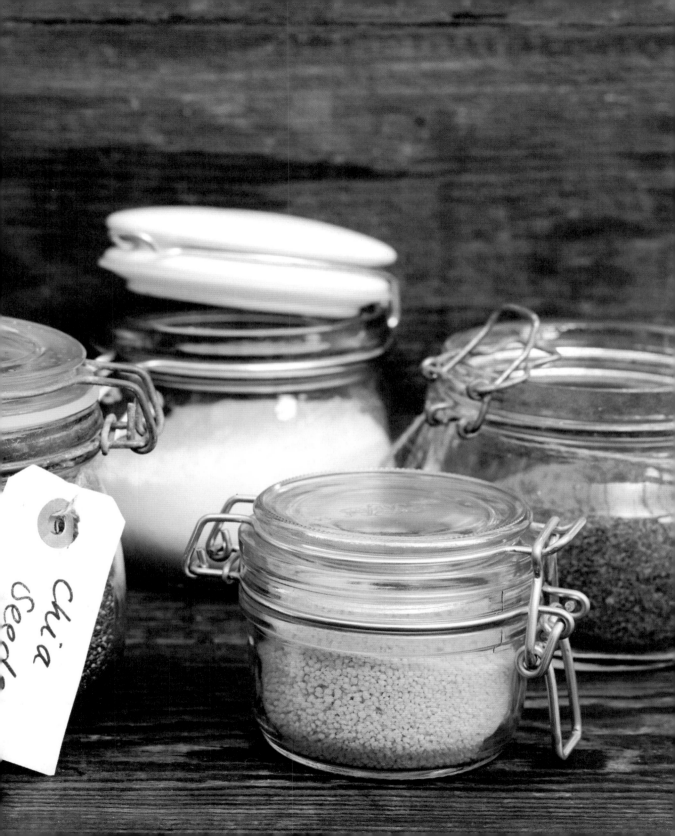

LUNCH

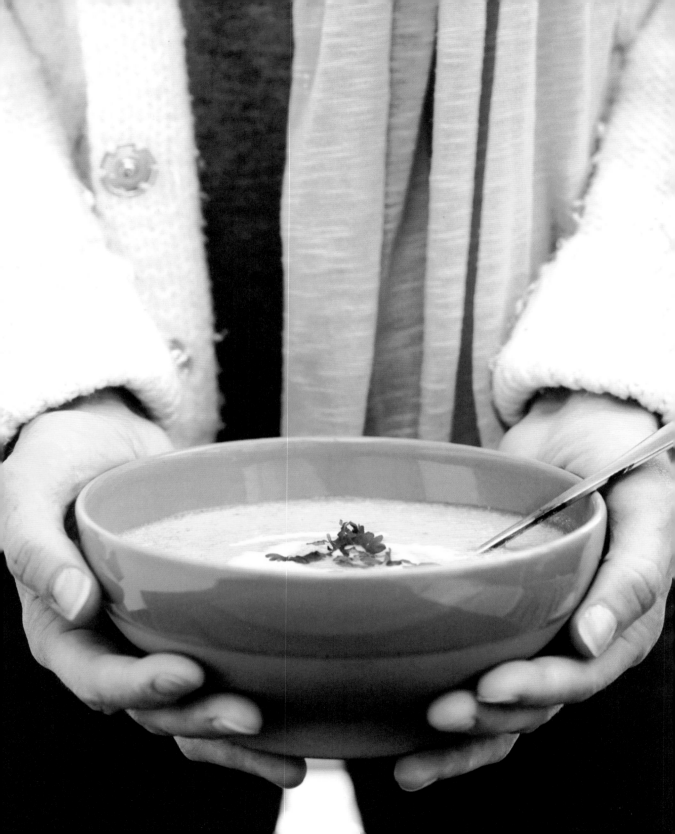

CHICKEN & VEGETABLE SOUP

Soup is so comforting and it's a great way to get nutritious food into you without much hassle. Some of my training sessions leave me completely knackered and it's always a relief to have a batch of this in the fridge ready to be heated up as I need it.

○ ○ ○○ ○○ ○ ○○ ○○ ○○ ○○ ○ ○○ ○○ ○○ ○○ ○ ○○ ○○ ○○ ○○ ○ ○○ ○○ ○○ ○○ ○ ○○ ○○ ○○ ○ ○○

SERVES 4

2 tbsp coconut oil

4 celery sticks, roughly chopped

2 carrots, peeled and roughly chopped

1 onion, roughly chopped

2 skinless chicken breast fillets, diced

2 potatoes, peeled and diced

2 sweet potatoes, peeled and diced

½ butternut squash, peeled, deseeded and diced

500ml chicken stock

1 tbsp dried mixed herbs

300ml milk

salt and pepper

Heat the coconut oil in a large pan over a medium heat. Add the celery, carrots and onion and cook for 10–15 minutes, until softened.

Add the chicken, potatoes, sweet potatoes, butternut, stock and herbs to the pot and bring to the boil. Reduce the heat, cover and simmer for 30 minutes.

Remove from the heat and stir in the milk. Purée with a hand blender until smooth. Season to taste and ladle the soup into warmed serving bowls.

STOCK

{ IN COOKERY SCHOOL WE HAD A GREAT CLASS ON MAKING FRESH STOCK. I TRY TO TAKE THE TIME TO DO THIS: THE FLAVOUR IS WORTH THE EFFORT. IF I DON'T HAVE TIME, I USE MARIGOLD SWISS VEGETABLE BOUILLON POWDER. }

CREAMY TOMATO & CANNELLINI BEAN SOUP

I love soup, and tomato is my favourite. I tried to grow tomatoes for the first time in 2012 and failed miserably, but I kept at it and grew some amazing ones in 2013. I grew them in the conservatory in big pots that sat beside my training weights! It looked rather odd but the tomatoes were happy to sit in with the weights. In the end, the tomatoes grew beautifully. I'm convinced that they're the fittest tomatoes in Ireland.

SERVES 2

2 tsp olive oil

1 onion, finely chopped

600g fresh whole tomatoes, quartered

½ red chilli, finely chopped

a pinch of salt

400g tin of chopped tomatoes

500ml vegetable stock

a handful of basil leaves

400g tin of cannellini beans, drained and rinsed

2 tsp cream, to serve

Heat the olive oil in a large pan over a medium heat. Add the onion and cook for about 5 minutes, until softened. Stir in the fresh tomatoes, chilli and salt. Cover and cook for 10 minutes, stirring occasionally.

Add the tinned tomatoes and stock to the pan and stir well. Cover and simmer for 20 minutes, stirring occasionally.

Take the pan off the heat and stir in the basil. Purée the soup with a hand blender until smooth. Stir in the cannellini beans. Return the pan to the heat and reheat gently. Ladle the soup into warmed serving bowls and top each one with a teaspoon of cream.

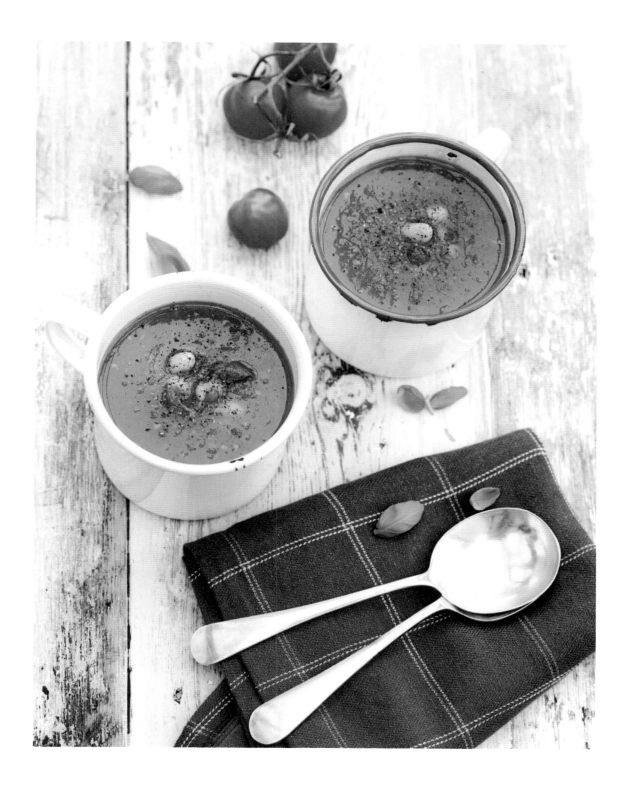

'TRUE STRENGTH OFTEN RISES
AT OUR WEAKEST POINT.'

EAMON FENNELL'S SOUP

Eamon was a player on the Dublin team that won the All-Ireland against Kerry in 2011. He's a super Gaelic footballer and in 2014 he lifted the All-Ireland trophy with his club, St Vincent's. I've spent time training in the gym with Eamon. He is so much fun to train with and most of the time our chats revolve around food. I like to tell him what I'm trying in the kitchen and he shares a few tips of his own. Eamon eats to perform well so he makes sure that he's well able to whip up healthy and tasty meals. Here is Eamon's recipe for a tasty soup.

SERVES 4

1 tbsp coconut oil

1 onion, finely chopped

3 garlic cloves, crushed

500g broccoli, broken into florets

1 sweet potato, peeled and diced

1 litre vegetable stock, plus extra if needed

1 tsp ground nutmeg

2 tbsp mascarpone

salt and pepper

Heat the coconut oil in a large pan over a medium heat. Add the onion and garlic and cook for 10 minutes, until softened.

Add the broccoli, sweet potato, stock and nutmeg to the pot and bring to the boil. Reduce the heat, cover and simmer for 30 minutes.

Remove from the heat and stir in the mascarpone. Purée with a hand blender until smooth. Season to taste and ladle the soup into warmed serving bowls.

SUPERFOOD SALAD

I don't have time to cook a superfood salad everyday but I still want to get my fix of healthy ingredients. Quinoa-based salads are the way to go. I cook a big batch of quinoa, let it cool and store it in the fridge in an airtight container. Then I use this as a base for loads of different superfood salads in the days that follow.

You can toast big batches of almonds or other nuts and stash them away. You can even prepare some of the fruit ahead of time. If you're chopping apples in advance, remember to squeeze over some lemon juice to keep them looking and tasting fresh.

o o o o o o o o o o o o o o o o o o o o o o o o o o o o o o o o o o o o o o o o

SERVES 1

a small bowl of cooked quinoa

1 tbsp toasted nuts, such as pine nuts,
    cashews or flaked almonds

1 piece of fruit, prepared, such as a
    chopped apple, a handful of
    blueberries or pomegranate seeds

a handful of leaves or raw vegetables,
    such as baby spinach or grated carrot

juice of ½ lemon or lime

3 tbsp olive oil

a handful of fresh herbs, such as basil,
    mint or parsley, chopped

2 tbsp mixed seeds, such as pumpkin
    and sunflower

a pinch of salt

1 tbsp Greek yoghurt, to garnish

Place all of the ingredients, except for the Greek yoghurt, in a serving bowl and mix well. Garnish with the Greek yoghurt and serve.

DESIRE IS WHAT GETS YOU STARTED.
HABIT IS WHAT KEEPS YOU GOING.

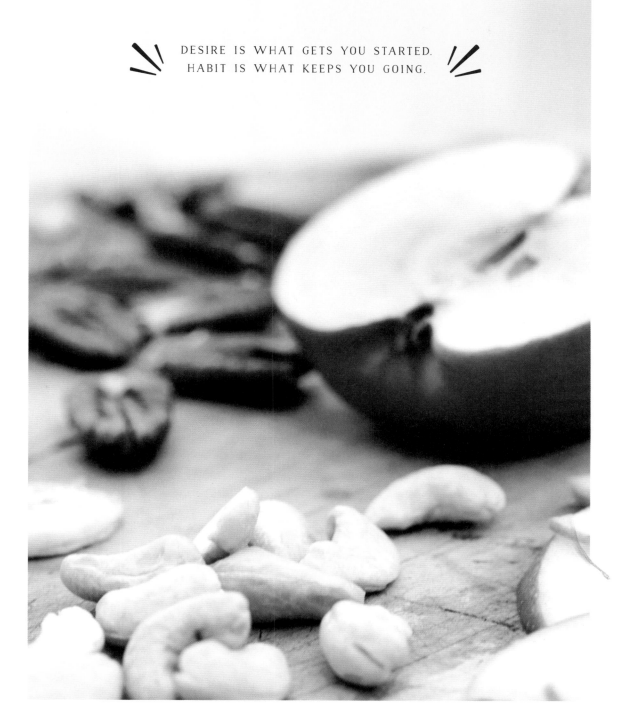

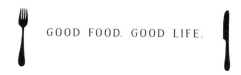

COCONUT &
CARROT SALAD

I love coconut. Anyone who doesn't like coconut makes me suspicious. I'm even partial

to the odd Bounty bar. Coconut adds lovely flavour and texture to this salad.

I eat this one a lot.

° °

SERVES 1

1 tsp agave syrup

a handful of coriander leaves

juice of 1 lime

2 small carrots, peeled and grated

salt

½ tsp coconut oil

½ tsp cumin seeds

50g desiccated coconut

Mix the agave syrup, coriander and lime juice in a large serving bowl. Add the grated carrots and a pinch of salt. Mix well to combine.

Heat the coconut oil in a large pan over a medium heat. Add the cumin seeds and cook for about 30 seconds, stirring all the time. Add the desiccated coconut and cook for 1–2 minutes, until golden. Remove the pan from the heat and leave to cool completely. Just before serving, tip the contents of the pan into the carrot mixture and stir well.

CHICKPEA & MANGO SALAD

This recipe makes two large portions and would be a perfect lunch when served with some Happy, Healthy Bread (p.135). The salad is also a great side dish for quinoa, baked fish or grilled meat. I like to make a double batch of the dressing because it keeps well in the fridge and gives me plenty of salad options in the days that follow.

SERVES 2

For the dressing

3 scallions, trimmed
½ mango, peeled and chopped
½ tsp paprika
3 tbsp olive oil
juice of 1 lime
a pinch of salt

For the salad

400g tin of chickpeas, drained
2 carrots, peeled and finely sliced
a handful of green beans, sliced
    crossways
2 tbsp finely chopped fresh
    coriander

Place all of the ingredients for the dressing in a food processor (or use a hand blender) and blitz until combined.

Place the chickpeas in a large serving bowl, tip in the mango dressing and stir to combine. Add the carrots and green beans and toss well. Sprinkle over the coriander and serve.

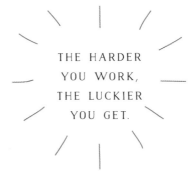

THE HARDER
YOU WORK,
THE LUCKIER
YOU GET.

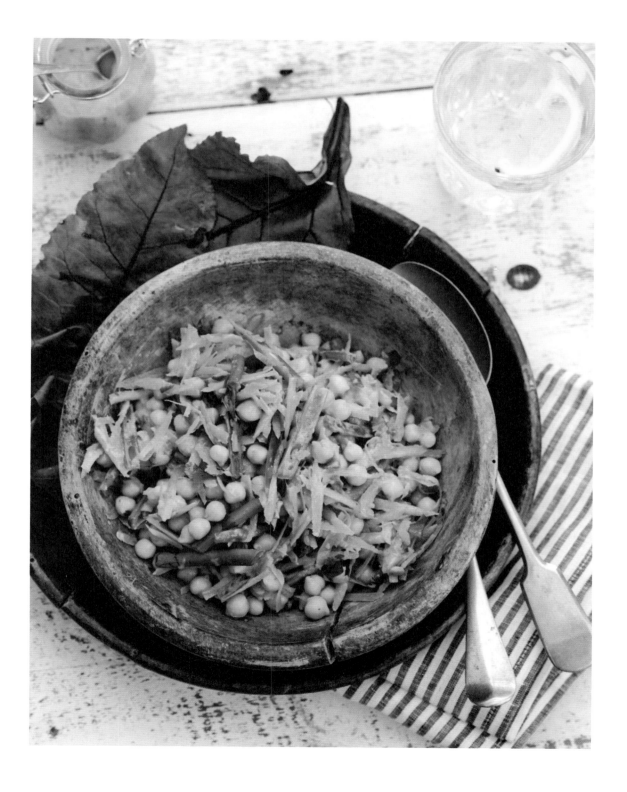

GREENS & QUINOA SALAD

This salad makes a tasty and healthy lunch. Sometimes I have it with tinned salmon or tuna for a fast nutritious meal. If I'm super-organised, which does happen sometimes, I have this with a cold salmon or chicken fillet that I've cooked the night before.

○ ○

SERVES 2

a handful of flaked almonds

170g quinoa, cooked and cooled

2 tbsp shop-bought sundried tomato pesto

2 handfuls of green beans, sliced crossways

2 handfuls of lettuce

a handful of basil leaves, chopped

a handful of coriander leaves

Preheat the oven to 180°C/350°F/gas 4. Spread the almonds on a baking tin and bake for 5–10 minutes or until toasted, turning halfway through. Set aside to cool.

Place the quinoa and pesto in a large serving bowl and stir well to combine. Add the green beans and lettuce and mix well. Scatter over the basil, coriander and toasted almonds. Serve without delay.

BEETROOT &
CARROT SALAD

It's always a good idea to reduce your consumption of processed foods. One piece of nutritional advice I hear a lot is to eat food as close as possible to its natural state. This can be a fairly tough ask, but salads like this one make it look easy.

Make sure to keep the beetroot and carrots apart until you're just about to serve. Grated beetroot has a strong colour that bleeds into other ingredients. It's much nicer if everything retains its own colour in this salad.

SERVES 4

3 beetroot, trimmed and peeled

3 carrots, peeled

2 tsp olive oil

4 shallots, finely chopped

1 tbsp cumin seeds

1½ tbsp red wine vinegar

a handful of mint leaves, chopped

2 tbsp sesame seeds or flaked almonds

Grate the beetroot and carrots in separate bowls and set aside.

Heat the olive oil in a large pan over a medium heat. Add the shallots and cook for about 10 minutes, until softened. Add the cumin seeds and cook for 3 minutes, stirring occasionally. Stir in the red wine vinegar, then take the pan off the heat.

Tip the contents of the pan into a large serving bowl. Stir in the grated beetroot and carrots. Add the mint and sesame seeds and stir well. Serve without delay.

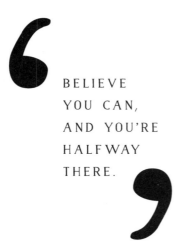

'BELIEVE
YOU CAN,
AND YOU'RE
HALFWAY
THERE.'

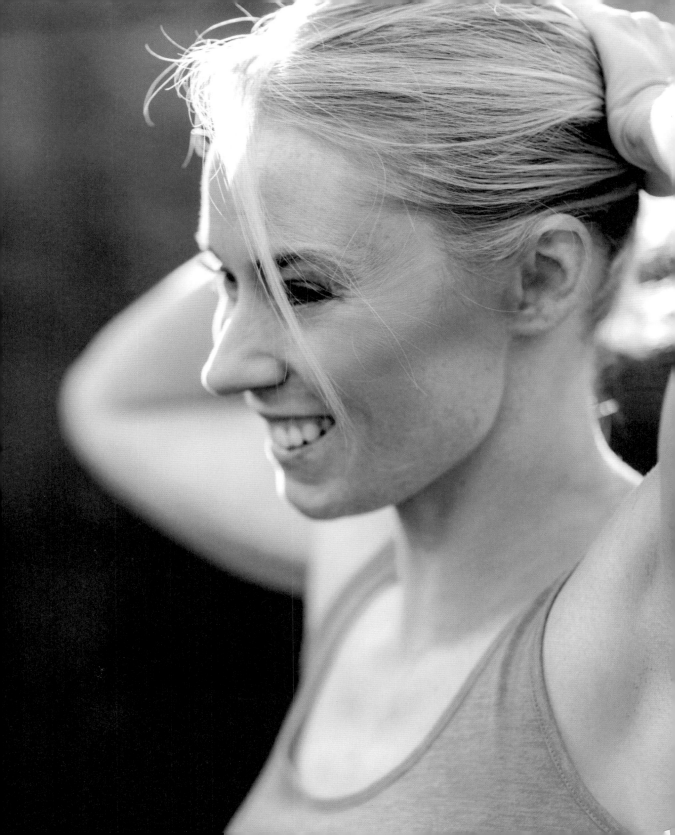

CHICKEN SALAD WITH BEETROOT, CARROT & QUINOA

Beetroot is a food I've only started eating in recent years. It seemed a bit inaccessible before, but now I love it. A lot of people juice beetroot but I like to work it into recipes so that I can eat it instead. For this salad, I prefer to let the chicken cool down but you don't have to – it's nice served warm too.

○ ○ ○○ ○ ○○ ○ ○ ○○ ○ ○ ○○ ○ ○ ○○ ○ ○ ○○ ○ ○ ○○ ○ ○ ○○ ○ ○ ○○ ○ ○ ○○ ○ ○ ○○ ○ ○ ○○ ○ ○ ○○ ○○ ○○

SERVES 4

100g quinoa
6 carrots, peeled and grated
2 beetroot, peeled and grated
3 tbsp olive oil
1 onion, finely chopped
2 tbsp cumin seeds
4 skinless chicken breast fillets
25g linseeds
50g sunflower seeds
150g Greek yoghurt
4 tbsp chopped fresh coriander

Cook the quinoa according to the instructions on the package and set aside to cool.

Combine the carrots and beetroot in a large mixing bowl. Heat the olive oil in a large frying pan over a medium heat. Add the onion and fry for about 10 minutes, until softened. Add the cumin seeds and cook for a further 2 minutes. Then tip the contents of the pan into the mixing bowl and stir well to combine.

Return the pan to the heat and cook the chicken fillets for about 5 minutes on each side, until golden and cooked through. Set aside to cool.

Meanwhile, add the linseeds, sunflower seeds and cooked quinoa to the carrot and beetroot salad. Stir until combined.

Stir the Greek yoghurt and coriander in a small mixing bowl.

Divide the salad between serving plates and arrange the cooked chicken on top. Add a dollop of the Greek yoghurt and coriander and serve.

WARM QUINOA WITH LEMON, PISTACHIO & HARISSA

This dish is full of bright, zingy and spicy flavours. I've often thrown it together in no time at all on a summer's day. Lemon. Pistachios. Spices. Glass of white wine. Summertime. Sold!

○ ○ ○○ ○○ ○○ ○○ ○○ ○ ○○ ○○ ○○ ○○ ○○ ○○ ○○ ○○ ○○ ○○ ○○ ○○ ○○ ○○ ○○ ○○ ○○ ○○ ○○

SERVES 1

1 tbsp coconut oil

2 carrots, peeled and diced

1 onion, peeled and finely chopped

3 garlic cloves, crushed

1 tsp ground cumin

1 tsp grated fresh ginger

½ tsp ground cinnamon

90g quinoa

500ml vegetable stock, simmering

½ tsp harissa

zest and juice of ½ lemon

a handful of coriander leaves

2 tbsp pistachios, crushed

Heat the coconut oil in a medium pan over a medium heat. Add the carrots and onions and cook for 10 minutes. Add the garlic, cumin, ginger and cinnamon and cook for a further 2 minutes. Add the quinoa and stock and stir well. Simmer, uncovered, for 15 minutes, stirring occasionally to ensure that the quinoa doesn't stick to the bottom of the pan.

Stir in the harissa and lemon juice (leaving aside the lemon zest). Spoon the cooked quinoa into a warmed serving bowl. Sprinkle over the lemon zest, coriander and pistachios and serve.

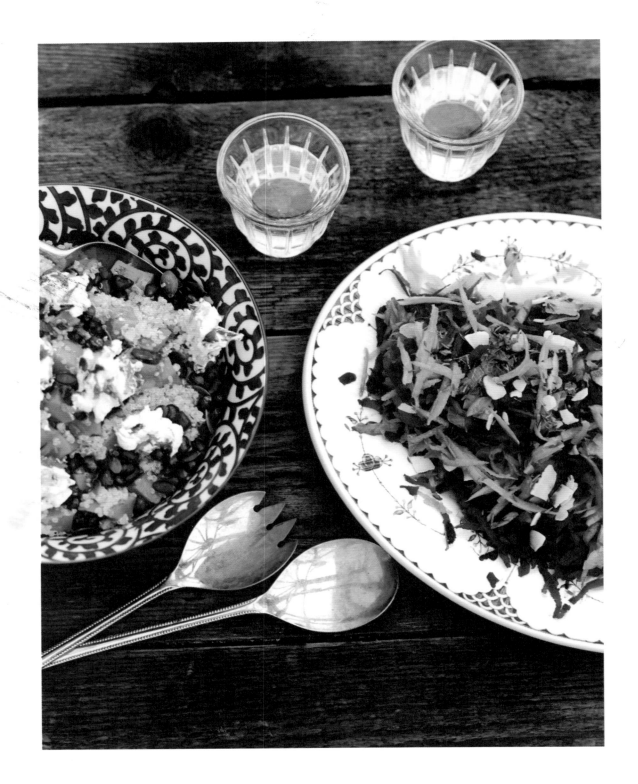

ROAST BUTTERNUT & QUINOA SALAD

This is a great salad because it is equally delicious served warm or cold. If you want to eat it cold, make a big batch of it and leave the butternut and quinoa to cool before assembling. This is a nice light lunch option but you could increase the portion if you wanted to eat it for dinner.

SERVES 4

½ butternut squash peeled, deseeded and cubed
olive oil
salt and pepper
2 garlic cloves, finely chopped
½ red chilli, finely chopped
170g quinoa or brown rice
50g goat's cheese
a handful of mint leaves, chopped
a handful of pumpkin seeds
½ pomegranate, seeds only

Preheat the oven to 180°C/350°F/gas 4.

Place the butternut cubes on a baking tray, drizzle with olive oil, season well and roast for 25 minutes. Remove from the oven and sprinkle over the garlic and chilli. Return to the oven for 5–10 minutes, until soft.

Meanwhile, cook the quinoa according to the instructions on the package.

Mix the roasted butternut and quinoa in a large bowl. Crumble in the goat's cheese, add the mint and stir well to combine. Divide the salad between serving plates. Sprinkle the pumpkin and pomegranate seeds over. Finish with a drizzle of olive oil and serve.

OATY CHICKEN STRIPS

These Oaty Chicken Strips are my idea of healthy chicken goujons. They make a gorgeous lunch if you have them with a big salad on the side. They could also be part of a very tasty dinner. And since they are marinated, they are tender and full of flavour.

○ ○ ○○

SERVES 4

4 tbsp soy sauce
2 tbsp olive oil
1 tsp dried oregano
1 tsp dried rosemary
1 tsp dried sage
1 tsp dried tarragon
a pinch of salt
4 skinless chicken breast fillets, cut into strips
60g porridge oats

Mix the soy sauce, olive oil, dried herbs and salt in a large bowl. Add the chicken and use your hands to massage the marinade into the meat. Cover and leave to marinate in the fridge for at least 1 hour.

Preheat the oven to 180°C/350°F/gas 4.

Spread the oats on a plate. Roll each chicken strip in the oats. Place the coated chicken strips in an ovenproof dish. Bake for about 30 minutes, until each chicken goujon is cooked through with a crispy coating.

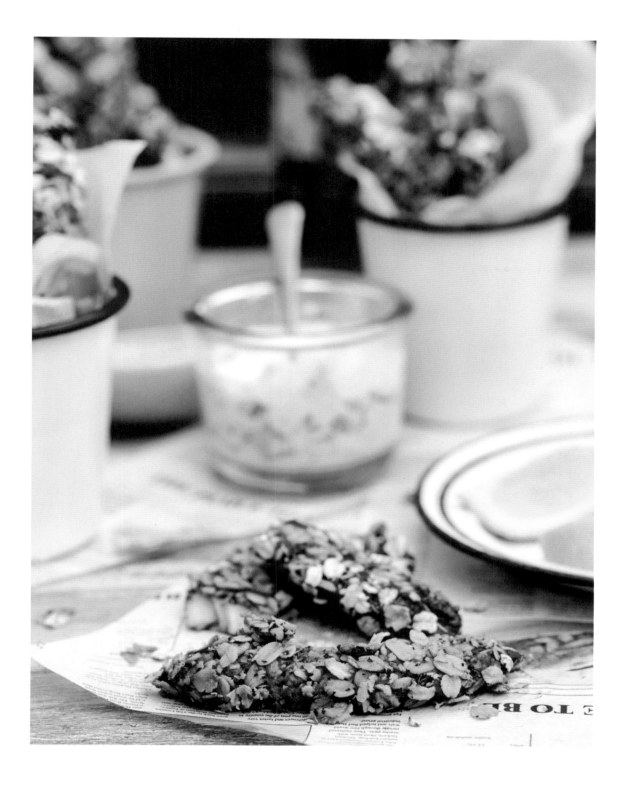

SUPPLEMENTS*

I don't believe there is any replacement for a good, healthy diet. But I do feel that supplements have their benefits and their place within a solid nutrition plan. I started taking supplements in my early twenties, after working out a plan with my nutritionist.

Before buying any supplement I ask myself a few questions. Is this product effective? Is it of high quality? Are the manufacturing practices assessed and maintained to a high standard? It is vital to be aware of what you are putting into your body. As always, careful reading of product labels is really important. As an athlete, I'm responsible for everything that's put into my body. I need to be extra vigilant to ensure that I comply with the anti-doping code.

I use products from certain companies, namely ROS Nutrition, USN and Kinetica. These companies tick all my boxes when it comes to standards and quality.

When I'm out and about or at the gym, many people ask me about the specific supplements I take. On the next page is a chart of my routine.

* Obviously, you have to be very careful when taking any supplements. Talk with your doctor or nutritionist. Watch out for companies or supplements that offer unrealistic results or promises. Don't fall for gimmicky marketing. Health and fitness cannot be built in a factory somewhere – they are created in your daily habits and in your kitchen!

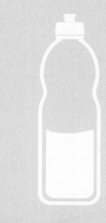

PRODUCT	WHEN I TAKE IT	WHY I TAKE IT
MULTIVITAMIN	Daily	To make sure I'm getting all of my nutrients
PROTEIN POWDER	Daily, during training phases	For growth and repair of lean tissue For adapting to training and repair from training
CARBOHYDRATE AND AMINO ACIDS DRINK	Daily after training sessions	To fuel and hydrate during training phases
ENERGY DRINK	During training sessions	To fuel and hydrate during training
FISH OILS	Daily	For omega-3 goodness

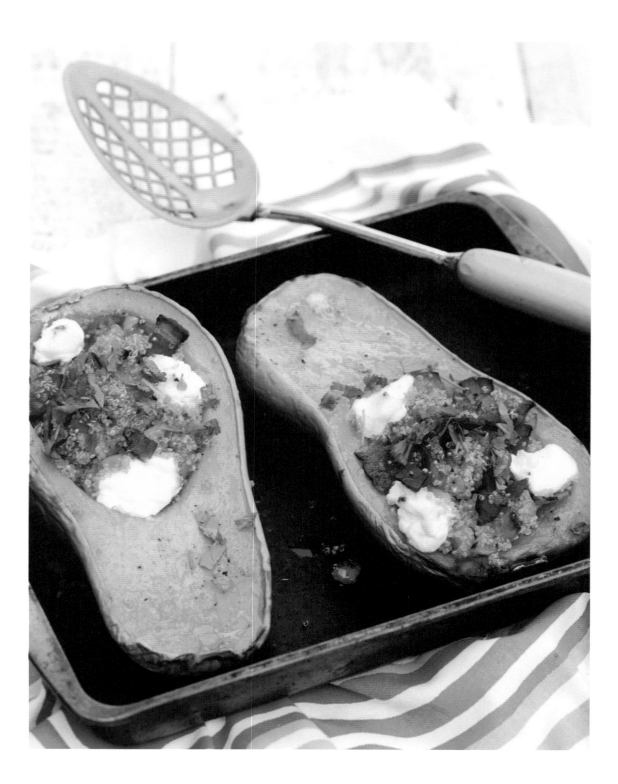

STUFFED BUTTERNUT

Butternut stays fresh for ages, so it's always a smart purchase. It scores well on the glycemic index too, so it will give you a slow release on energy. This recipe is butternut with a bit of bling.

∘ ∘ ∘∘

SERVES 2 SMALL PORTIONS

1 butternut squash (a short and stout one,
    rather than a long and slim one)
1 tsp olive oil
2 peppers, finely chopped
½ onion, finely chopped
4 pancetta slices or 3 rashers, thinly sliced
100g cooked quinoa
40g goat's cheese

Preheat the oven to 180°C/350°F/gas 4.

Cut the butternut in half lengthways and scoop out the pips. Place the butternut halves in an ovenproof dish and roast for 30 minutes.

Meanwhile, heat the olive oil in a medium pan over a medium heat. Cook the peppers and onion for 10 minutes. Add the pancetta and cook for 3 minutes. Remove from the heat, stir in the cooked quinoa and set aside.

Carefully remove the butternut halves from the oven and spoon the quinoa mixture into them. Crumble over the goat's cheese and return the butternut halves to the oven for 15 minutes. Once the filling has heated through and the goat's cheese has melted, the Stuffed Butternut is ready to serve.

DAVID GILLICK'S FRITTATA

David was double European Indoor Champion. The first time he won gold I was sitting in an ice-bath screaming at the TV watching him! It was a huge breakthrough for an Irish athlete to win a sprint medal and David's performance totally inspired me. I wanted to win medals too.

I've travelled all over the world with David. I've had dinner with him in Japan. I've had wine with him in Barcelona on his birthday after he ran 44 seconds and won a meet there. I've dragged him to McDonald's in small towns all over Europe to eat McFlurrys and talk about the races we just ran. David and I have been through all the highs and lows of high-performance athletics together.

The best athletes learn how to cook – because if you want to run fast, you need to fuel yourself really well. David is a great cook. He won Celebrity MasterChef Ireland in 2013. It's a cool combination: a guy who can run 400 metres in 44 seconds and who is handy in the kitchen. Here is David's recipe for a frittata.

SERVES 2

60g quinoa, cooked and cooled

4 eggs (2 whole eggs, plus 2 egg whites)

salt and pepper

paprika

1 tsp coconut oil

70g bacon, finely sliced

½ onion, finely chopped

1 small pepper, finely chopped

80g mushrooms, finely chopped

100g tinned chopped tomatoes

Preheat the grill to a high heat.

Lightly beat the eggs in a medium bowl. Season and add paprika to taste.

Heat the coconut oil in a large ovenproof frying pan over a medium-high heat. Cook the bacon, onion, pepper and mushrooms for about 10 minutes. Add the cooked quinoa and chopped tomatoes and stir well.

Reduce to a low heat and pour the eggs into the pan. Do not stir the eggs: use a wooden spoon to move the ingredients around and allow the eggs to leak into any available gaps. Cook for about 10 minutes, until the frittata is softly set and golden underneath. Place the frying pan under the preheated grill for a few minutes, until the top of the frittata is set and golden.

Cut the frittata into slices and serve on warmed plates.

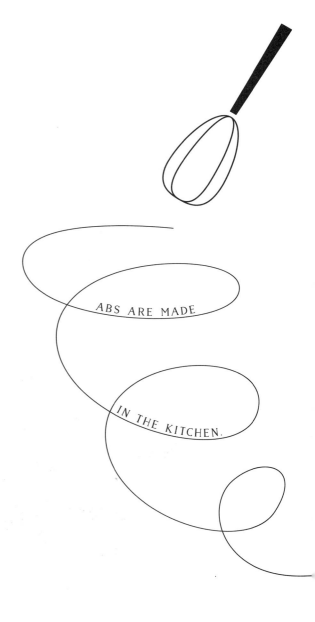

ABS ARE MADE IN THE KITCHEN.

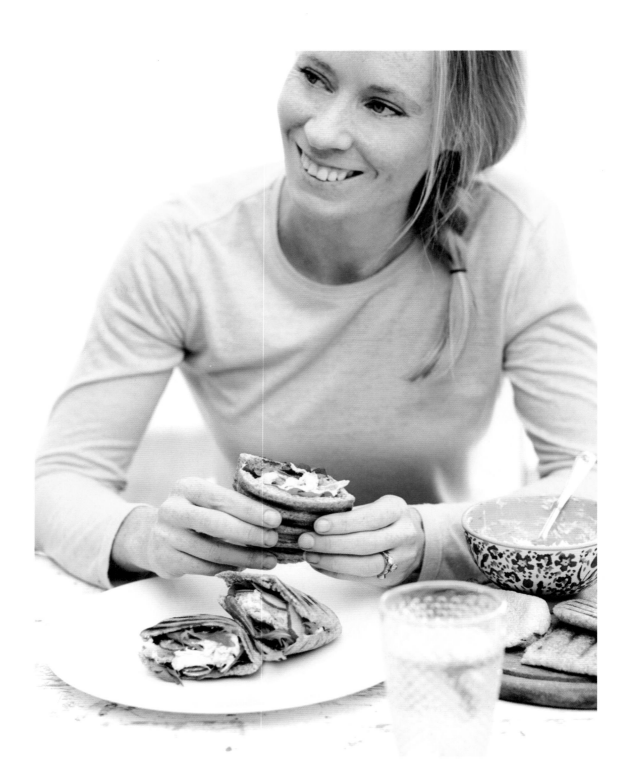

SPICY CHICKEN PITTA

I like to eat nutritious food and I believe that there is just no excuse for a boring sambo. Chicken and curry make a classic combination. This is a speedy, tasty and healthy lunch.

○ ○ ○○

SERVES 1

1 tsp coconut oil

1 skinless chicken breast fillet, diced

2 tbsp flaked almonds

2 tbsp natural yoghurt

1 tsp curry powder

½ tsp cinnamon

½ tsp turmeric

1 wholemeal pitta

1 carrot, grated

a small handful of rocket leaves

Melt the coconut oil in a small pan over a medium heat and cook the chicken for about 5 minutes, until golden and cooked through. Set aside to cool slightly.

Mix the almonds, yoghurt, curry powder, cinnamon and turmeric in a small bowl. Add the cooked chicken and stir well.

Quickly toast the pitta on both sides. Split open and stuff with the chicken mixture, carrot and rocket. Serve without delay.

SALMON AND DILL PITTA: is another favourite lunch of mine. Mix these ingredients in a small bowl: • 1 salmon fillet, cooked and chopped • 1 tbsp Greek yoghurt • 1 tsp dill (fresh or dried) • 1 tsp lemon juice. Then toast the pitta, stuff it and enjoy!

LUNCHTIME FRITTATA

Eggs are the perfect food: they are so nutritious and super-versatile. That's why they really can be an athlete's best friend! What other food could you have for breakfast, lunch and dinner?

o o o o o o o o o o o o o o o o o o o o o o o o o o o o o o o o o o o o o o o o o o o

SERVES 3

6 eggs
2 tbsp freshly chopped herbs, such as basil, coriander and parsley
1 tbsp cream cheese
1 tbsp Cheddar, grated
salt and pepper
1 tbsp coconut oil
1 small leek, finely chopped
1 small pepper, finely chopped
6 cherry tomatoes, halved

Preheat the grill to a high heat.

Lightly beat the eggs in a medium bowl. Add the herbs, cream cheese and Cheddar and season to taste.

Heat the coconut oil in a large ovenproof frying pan over a medium-high heat. Cook the leek and pepper for about 10 minutes.

Reduce to a low heat and pour the eggs into the pan. Do not stir the eggs: use a wooden spoon to move the ingredients around and allow the eggs to leak into any available gaps. Cook for about 10 minutes.

Meanwhile, place the tomato halves in an ovenproof dish under the preheated grill. Cook for about 5 minutes, until the tomatoes are warmed and softened.

When the frittata is softly set and golden underneath, remove the pan from the heat. Arrange the grilled tomatoes on top of the frittata in the pan. Place the pan under the grill for a few minutes and cook until the top of the frittata is set and golden.

Cut the frittata into slices and serve on warmed plates.

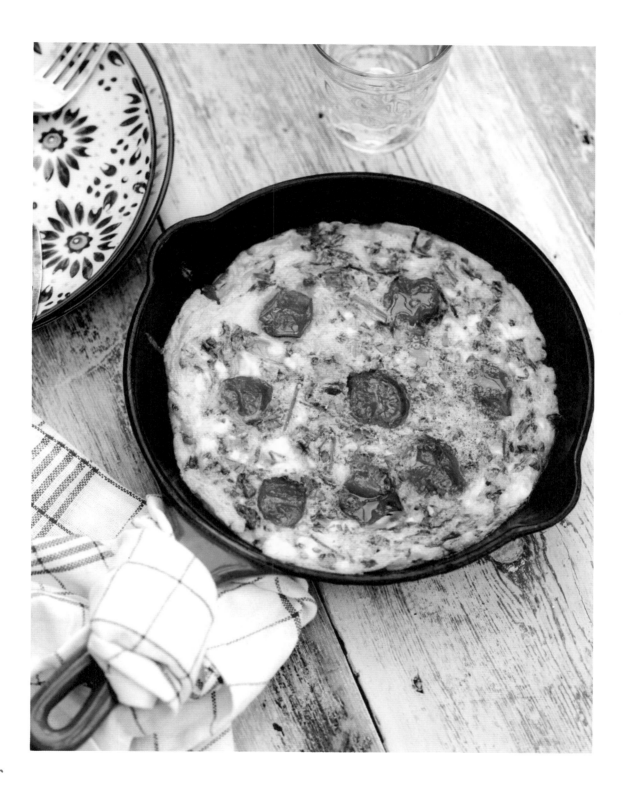

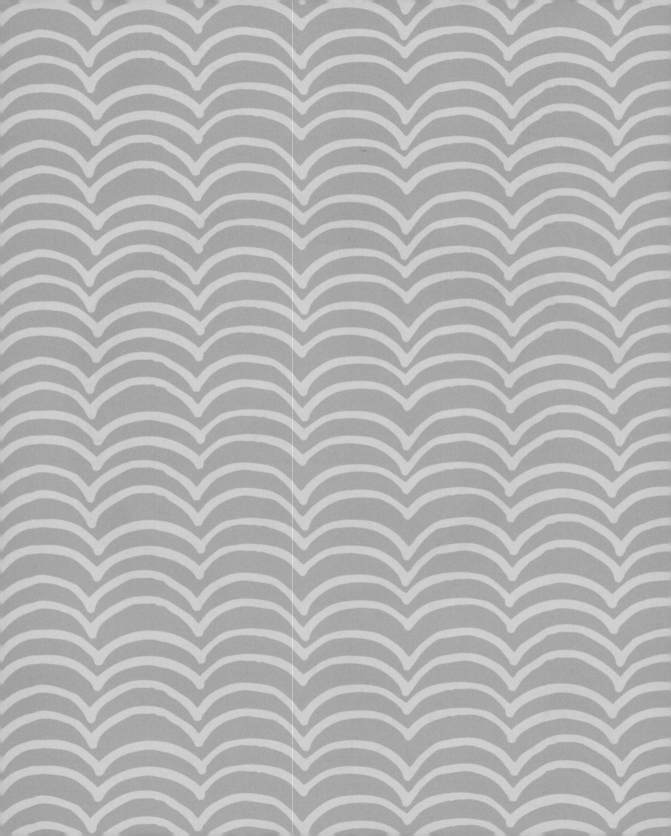

DINNER

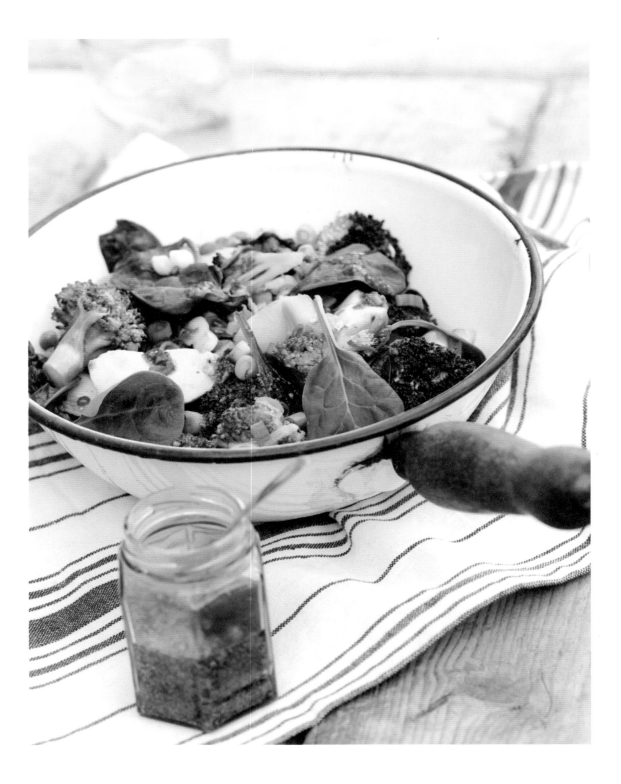

PESTO SPRING CHICKEN

This is a one-pot casserole that is perfect for spring. It's quick and easy and it warms you up on colder days. Sometimes, if I'm feeling very organised, I pre-cook this recipe to a certain stage and then stash it in the freezer. So when I come home after a busy day I can heat it through and add the vegetables – and dinner is done.

○ ○ ○ ○

SERVES 2

1 tbsp olive oil

3 shallots, finely chopped

2 skinless chicken breast fillets, quartered

3 medium-sized potatoes, peeled and halved

500ml vegetable stock

200g broccoli, broken into small florets

200g scallions, finely sliced

150g frozen peas

a handful of baby spinach

2 tbsp basil pesto

salt and pepper

Heat the olive oil in a large casserole over a medium heat. Add the shallots and cook for about 10 minutes, until softened. Add the chicken and cook for 5 minutes. Add the potatoes and stock and bring to the boil. Reduce the heat and simmer for 30 minutes.

If you want to pre-cook this casserole, now is the time to take it off the heat. Let it cool fully before storing it in an airtight container in the freezer.

Add the broccoli, scallions, peas and spinach to the casserole and cook for 5 minutes. Add the basil pesto and stir well. Check the seasoning and ladle the casserole into warmed serving bowls.

CHICKEN & LENTIL CASSEROLE

This recipe is pure comfort food and turkey is another lean meat that works really well here. Ideally, you should marinate the meat for an hour but don't worry if you don't have all that time (I rarely do). A little marinating is better than none.

○ ○

SERVES 4

2 garlic cloves, crushed

1 tbsp ground coriander

1 tbsp ground cumin

1 tsp paprika

4 skinless chicken breast fillets

2 tbsp olive oil

1 onion, finely chopped

100g chorizo, sliced into 2cm rounds

400g tin of chopped tomatoes

100g dried apricots, chopped

50g split red lentils

1 cinnamon stick

200ml water

a handful of flaked almonds

a handful of mint leaves, chopped

brown rice, to serve

Mix the garlic, coriander, cumin and paprika in a large bowl. Add the chicken and use your hands to massage the marinade into the meat. Cover and leave to marinate in the fridge for 1 hour.

Preheat the oven to 180°C/350°F/gas 4.

Heat the olive oil in a large casserole over a medium heat. Add the onion and chorizo and cook for about 10 minutes. Add the tomatoes, apricots, lentils, cinnamon stick, water and marinated chicken and stir well. Cover the casserole and place it in the oven for 1½ hours.

Meanwhile, spread the almonds on a baking tin and bake for 5–10 minutes or until toasted, turning halfway through.

Ladle the cooked casserole into warmed serving bowls and sprinkle over the almonds and mint. Serve with brown rice.

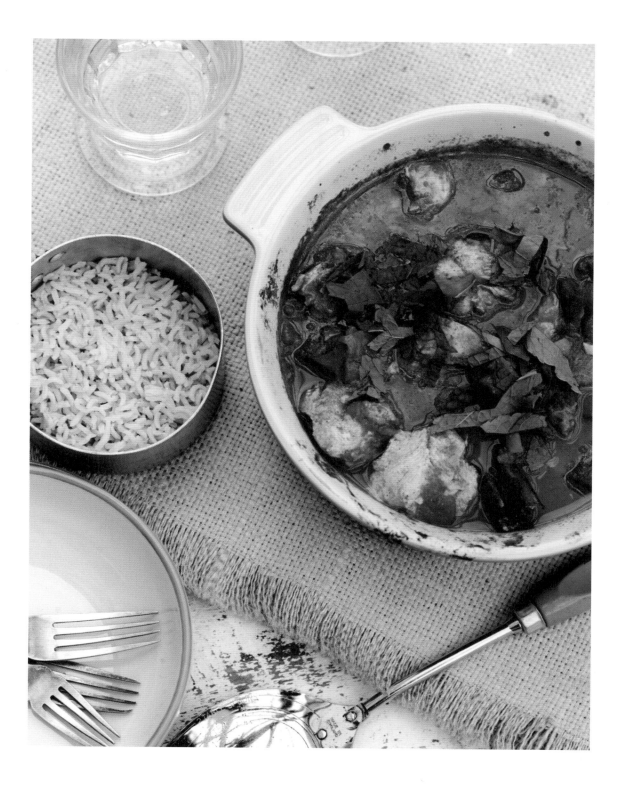

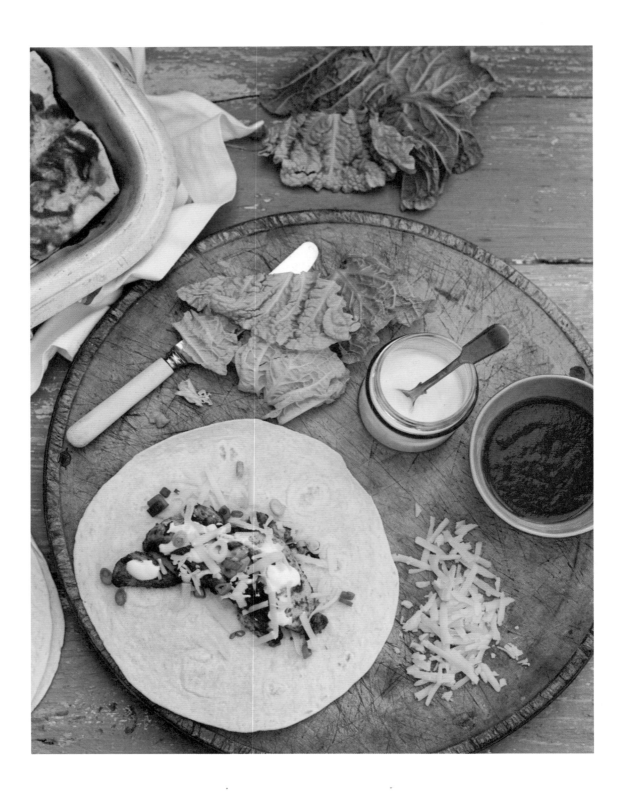

ENCHILADAS

Enchiladas are great for lunch or dinner. I'll confess that I've sometimes made a double batch of this at lunchtime so that I could eat it for dinner as well. Having the same lunch and dinner is not ideal – but when you're very busy and still want something healthy and tasty, go for it!

○ ○

SERVES 2

1 ripe avocado, peeled and cubed

a handful of mint leaves, chopped

juice of 1 lime

2 tbsp olive oil

½ red onion, finely chopped

2 skinless chicken breast fillets, cubed

2 tbsp fajita spice mix (homemade or shop-bought)

1 garlic clove, crushed

2 tortilla wraps

60ml tomato passata

50g Cheddar, grated

2 tbsp Greek yoghurt, to serve

brown rice, to serve (optional)

Preheat the oven to 180°C/350°F/gas 4.

Use a fork to mash the avocado, mint and lime juice in a small bowl and set aside.

Heat the olive oil in a large pan over a medium heat. Add the onion and cook for about 10 minutes, until softened. Add the chicken, spice mix and garlic and cook for 3–5 minutes, then set aside.

Divide the avocado mixture between the two tortillas, spreading it into an even layer. Add a layer of passata, followed by a layer of the spicy chicken mixture. Neatly roll each tortilla, then place them side by side in an ovenproof dish. Sprinkle the Cheddar over and place in the oven. Bake for 15–20 minutes.

Divide the enchiladas between warmed serving plates and top each one with a dollop of Greek yoghurt. Serve the brown rice on the side.

CHICKEN, BROCCOLI & QUINOA BAKE

This makes a tasty dinner and the leftovers are great for lunch the next day. If I want to make it more substantial, I serve it with a baked potato or some Sweet Potato Mash. Even by itself, it's lovely comfort food and it's so much better for you than gloopy, cheesy pasta bakes.

○ ○ ○○

SERVES 4

350g Greek yoghurt
1 tbsp curry powder
2 tsp gram or plain flour
1 tsp Dijon mustard
Juice of ½ lemon
180g quinoa, cooked and cooled
4 skinless chicken breast fillets, cooked, cooled
    and shredded
300g broccoli, cooked and cooled
salt
30g Parmesan, grated
30g pine nuts
Sweet Potato Mash (p.122), to serve (optional)

Preheat the oven to 160°C/325°F/gas 3.

Mix the Greek yoghurt, curry powder, gram flour, mustard and lemon juice in a small bowl and set aside.

Spread the cooked quinoa in an even layer in the base of an ovenproof dish. Mix the chicken, broccoli and a pinch of salt in a medium bowl, and arrange this mixture in another layer on top of the quinoa. Pour the Greek yoghurt mixture into the dish, spreading it into an even layer, and sprinkle the Parmesan and pine nuts over. Bake for about 40 minutes. Divide the bake between warmed serving bowls and serve with Sweet Potato Mash.

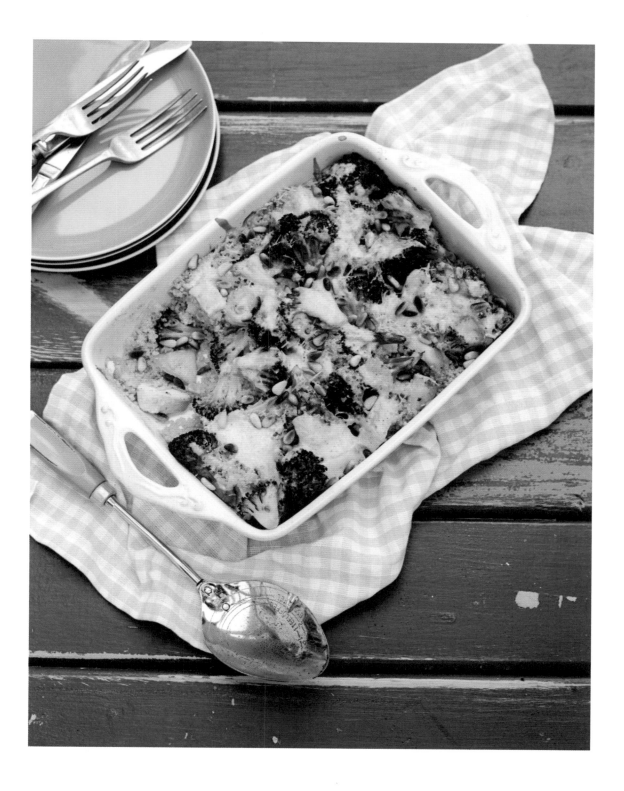

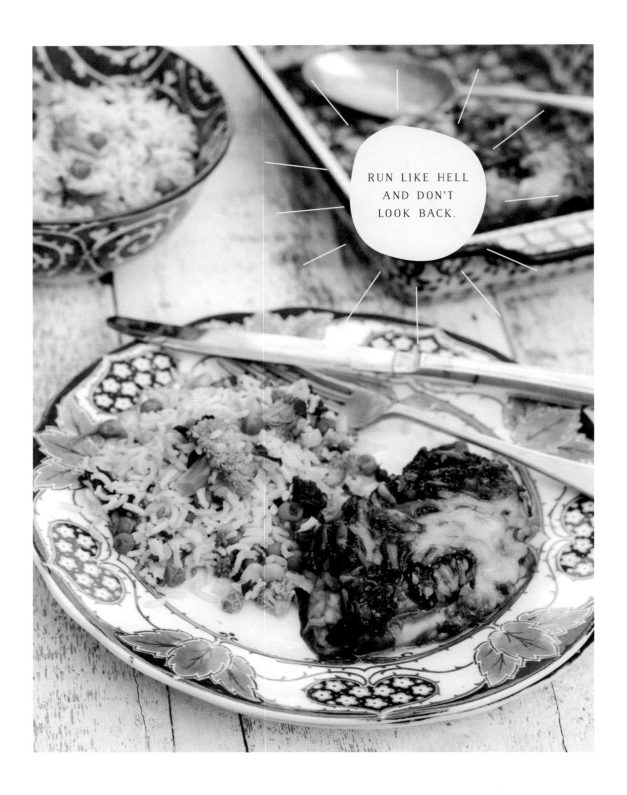

RUN LIKE HELL
AND DON'T
LOOK BACK.

SUPER-FAST CHICKEN & RICE

This dish is one that I cook when I am so tired from training that there is no chance of me making anything that takes major effort. I like having a few meals like this in my repertoire. This dinner is not as healthy as some of my other recipes but it definitely hits the spot after a track session and, all in all, it's not a bad option to throw together.

○ ○ ○○

SERVES 2

salt and pepper

2 skinless chicken breast fillets

2 tbsp Dijon mustard

2 tbsp chutney (plum, mango or whatever's in the cupboard)

a small handful of grated Cheddar

125g brown rice

300g mixed frozen vegetables

Preheat the oven to 180°C/350°F/gas 4.

Season the chicken fillets and place them in an ovenproof dish. Mix the Dijon mustard and chutney in a small bowl and coat the chicken fillets with this mixture. Sprinkle over the Cheddar. Bake the chicken for about 20 minutes, until cooked through.

Meanwhile, prepare the rice according to the instructions on the package.

About 5 minutes before serving, boil the vegetables in salted water, until tender.

Arrange the chicken on warmed serving plates and serve the rice and vegetables on the side.

SPICY TURKEY WRAPS

This is a recipe I turn to when I need to get away from starchy foods. Using Little Gem lettuce leaves as wraps is a great way to make a light and refreshing lunch.

○ ○

SERVES 2

2 red peppers, deseeded and finely sliced

1 small carrot, grated

⅓ cucumber, deseeded and diced

2 tbsp raw cashews, chopped

a handful of coriander leaves

250g turkey mince

4 scallions, finely sliced

2 garlic cloves, crushed

1 small red chilli, deseeded and finely sliced

a thumb-sized piece of ginger, grated

salt

1 tbsp coconut oil

2 heads of Little Gem lettuce, leaves
    separated, to serve

For the dressing

2 tbsp soy sauce

1 tsp agave syrup

½ tsp Tabasco sauce (or ½ chilli, deseeded
    and finely chopped)

juice of 1 lime

Toss the peppers, carrot, cucumber, cashews and coriander in a large bowl and set aside.

Combine the turkey mince, scallions, garlic, chilli, ginger and a pinch of salt in a large bowl. Heat the coconut oil in a large pan over a medium-high heat and cook the turkey mixture for about 10 minutes. Then drain any excess water from the turkey mixture.

Meanwhile, place all of the ingredients for the dressing in a jar with a lid and shake to combine.

Add the cooked turkey to the salad mix. Drizzle the dressing on top and toss well to combine.

Fill the lettuce leaves with spoonfuls of the turkey mix and serve immediately.

EATING OUT

I'm a healthy girl but let's be honest: life would be seriously boring if we didn't get to eat out every now and again. I love to go out for food – it's my very favourite social activity. Eating out is part of my life, anyway: I spend loads of time travelling and I end up eating in restaurants all over the world at track meets. Over the years, I've learned a few tricks so that I can eat out, mind my health and still have a great time.

Drink water instead of fizzy drinks.

Choose wholemeal bread for your sandwich.

If you don't cook a lot of fish at home, take your opportunity to eat some delicious fish in a restaurant.

Choose a salad as your side dish – and ask for the dressing to be served separately.

Choose lean meats, such as chicken or turkey.

Order main dishes that include vegetables (stir-fries are great).

Try broths and tomato-based sauces: they are usually healthier than creamy sauces.

Choose steamed or grilled dishes, rather than fried or sautéed dishes.

Before you order, look at the portion sizes that are being served. If a main dish looks way bigger than what you would normally eat, order two starters instead.

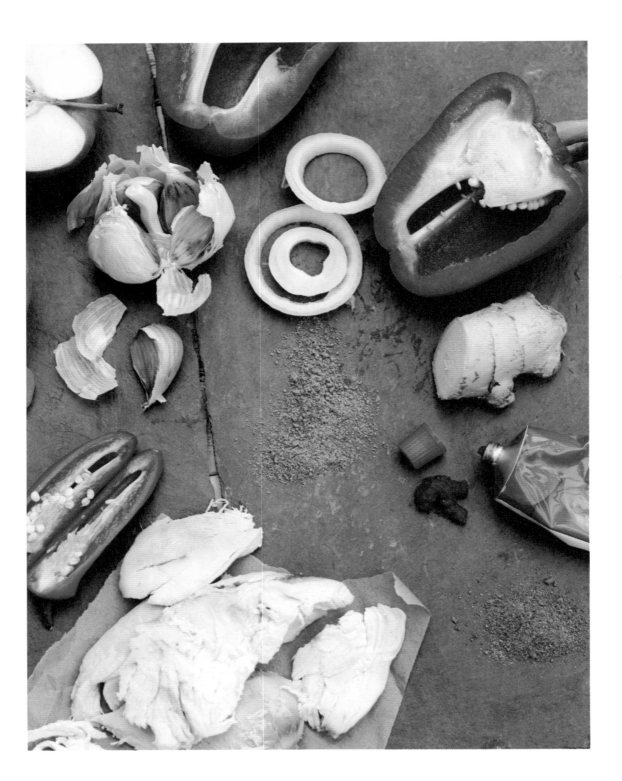

SIMPLE CURRY

Whenever I've a heavy training schedule coming up, I need to think carefully about my diet. If I know I will be spending three hours in the gym every day, I also know I won't be in the mood to cook a new dinner every night. Planning is essential and this curry is a basic recipe I know I can rely on. I often make a big batch of the curry sauce and freeze it in portions. Then all I need to do is heat through the sauce, stir in some cooked chicken or turkey – and dinner is sorted.

SERVES 4

3 tbsp coconut oil

2 onions, roughly chopped

4–5 garlic cloves, crushed

a thumb-sized piece of ginger, grated

2 tbsp medium curry powder

1 tsp garam masala

1 tsp ground coriander

½ tsp chilli flakes

10 dried apricots, halved

3 apples, peeled and roughly chopped

3 peppers, deseeded and roughly chopped

2 tbsp tomato purée

700ml chicken stock

salt and pepper

4 chicken or turkey breasts, cooked and shredded, to serve

brown or basmati rice, to serve

Heat the coconut oil in a large pot over a medium heat. Add the onions and cook for about 10 minutes, until softened. Add the garlic, ginger and spices and fry for 3 minutes, stirring occasionally. Stir in the apricots, apples, peppers, tomato purée and chicken stock and bring to the boil. Reduce the heat, cover and simmer for at least 40 minutes (up to 60 minutes, if you have time).

If you want to pre-cook this curry, now is the time to take it off the heat. Let it cool fully, divide it into portions in airtight containers and store it in the freezer.

Use a hand blender to purée the curry sauce to the desired consistency, then check the seasoning.

Stir in the cooked chicken or turkey. When the curry is piping hot, ladle it into warmed serving bowls. Serve with brown or basmati rice.

ROAST CHICKEN

I love roast chicken. It's so easy to pop it in the oven and then, a little while later, you come back and there it is in all its tastiness. Even though this recipe serves four people, you don't need to have four people in the house if you want to make it! Roast chicken is brilliant for leftovers – it's a perfect base for lunches during the week.

∘ ∘

SERVES 4

olive oil

a small bunch of thyme

2 lemons, sliced

salt

1 x 1.5kg–2kg free-range chicken

6 potatoes, peeled

Preheat the oven to 180°C/350°F/gas 4.

Drizzle some olive oil in a large roasting tin or ovenproof dish. Arrange the thyme and lemon slices in a layer in the roasting tin. Sprinkle over some salt and place the chicken on top of this. Loosely cover the roasting tin with foil (to keep the chicken moist while it cooks).

Place the chicken in the oven and roast according to weight: 20 minutes per pound (454g) plus 10–20 minutes extra.

About 40 minutes from the end, add the potatoes to the roasting tin. For the final 10 minutes of cooking, remove the tinfoil so that the chicken gets a golden colour.

Leave the chicken to rest for at least 20 minutes before serving.

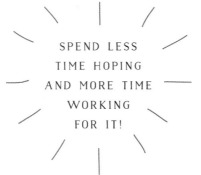

SPEND LESS
TIME HOPING
AND MORE TIME
WORKING
FOR IT!

ON THE SIDE: These yummy sides go really well with Roast Chicken:
• Carrots & Oats (p.120) • Red Cabbage & Apple (p.120) • Sweet Potato Mash (p.122)

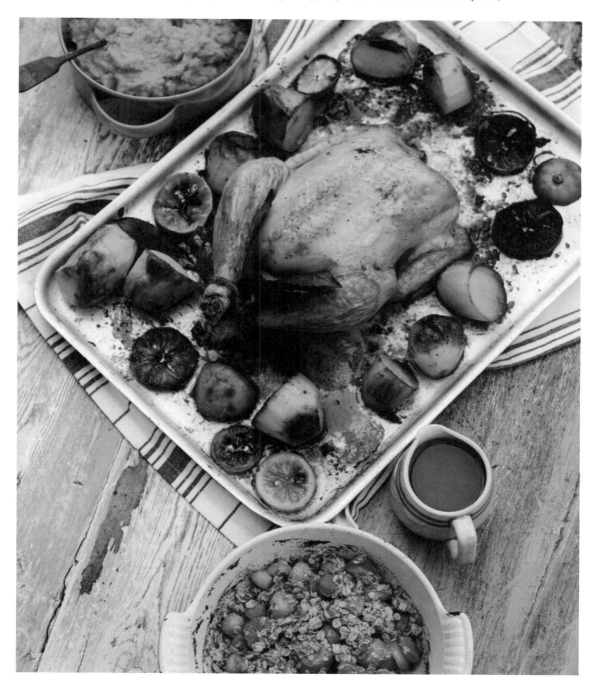

QUICK COCONUT & BASIL CHICKEN

This recipe combines lovely flavours. You can make it really quickly, so it's perfect for those nights when you don't want to spend too long cooking but still want to eat something healthy and tasty.

○ ○ ○○

SERVES 2

2 tbsp olive oil

4 shallots, finely sliced

2 leeks, trimmed and finely sliced

1 red chilli, deseeded and finely chopped

2 skinless chicken breast fillets, cubed

1 tbsp fish sauce

1 tsp agave syrup

a handful of basil leaves, torn

300ml coconut milk

brown or basmati rice, to serve

Heat the olive oil in a large pan over a medium heat. Add the shallots, leeks and chilli and cook for about 10 minutes. If the pan gets too dry, add a dash of water.

Add the chicken and cook for about 5 minutes, stirring often. Add the fish sauce, agave syrup, basil and coconut milk to the chicken in the pan. Stir well and cook for 2–3 minutes.

Serve piping hot in warmed serving bowls along with some brown or basmati rice.

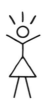

SHE WOKE UP ONE DAY

AND

THREW

AWAY

ALL

HER

EXCUSES

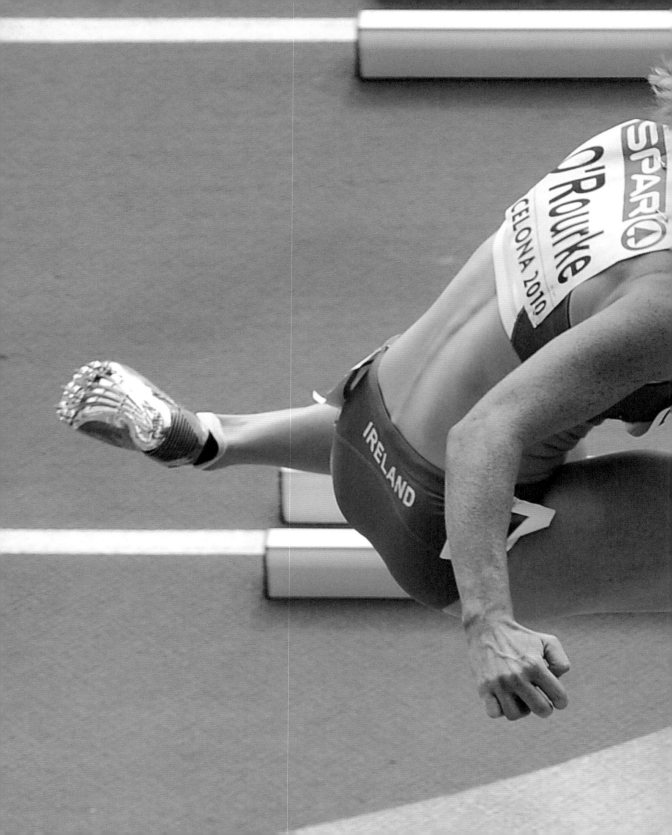

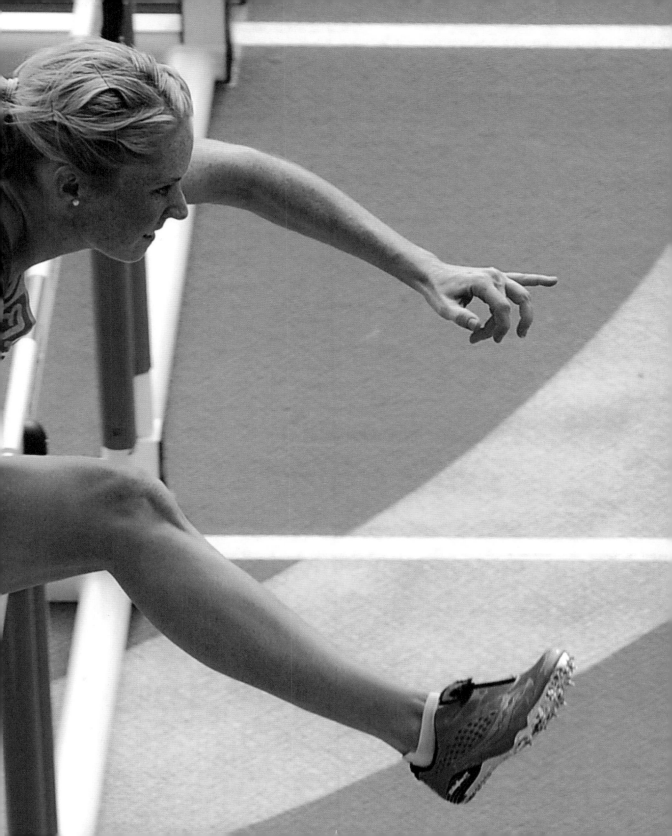

THAI RED CURRY

I use chicken and butternut here but this is a very flexible recipe, so feel free to adapt. During busy training periods, I often make a double batch of this curry because it tastes great on the second day. While it is a good idea to cook this curry in advance, it is never a good idea to cook rice in advance. Reheated rice can cause food poisoning – not good for the training schedule. Food poisoning is definitely in the Top Five Fears of Athletes!

○○ ○○

SERVES 2

1 tbsp coconut oil

1 onion, finely chopped

½ tsp ground ginger or 1 tsp grated
   fresh ginger

1 garlic clove, crushed

1 tbsp Thai red curry paste (2 tbsp for
   medium heat)

400ml tin of coconut milk

½ butternut squash peeled, deseeded
   and cubed

2 skinless chicken breast fillets, cubed

125g brown rice

3 cardamom pods

2 bay leaves

1 cinnamon stick

a handful of flaked almonds

juice of ½ lime

a handful of coriander leaves,
   chopped

Preheat the oven to 150°C/300°F/gas 2.

Melt the coconut oil in a large pan over a medium heat. Add the onion and ginger and cook for about 10 minutes, until softened. Add the garlic and curry paste and cook for 1–2 minutes, stirring all the time. Pour in the coconut milk and bring to the boil. Add the butternut and simmer, uncovered, for about 15 minutes. Add the chicken and stir well. Simmer, uncovered, for about 12 minutes, stirring occasionally.

Meanwhile, cook the rice according to the instructions on the package, adding the cardamom pods, bay leaves and cinnamon stick to the cooking water.

Spread the almonds on a baking tin and bake for about 10 minutes or until toasted, turning halfway through.

Before serving, add the lime juice and coriander to the curry and stir well. Spoon the cooked rice into warmed serving bowls, making a well in the centre. Ladle the curry on top of the rice, garnish with the toasted almonds and serve.

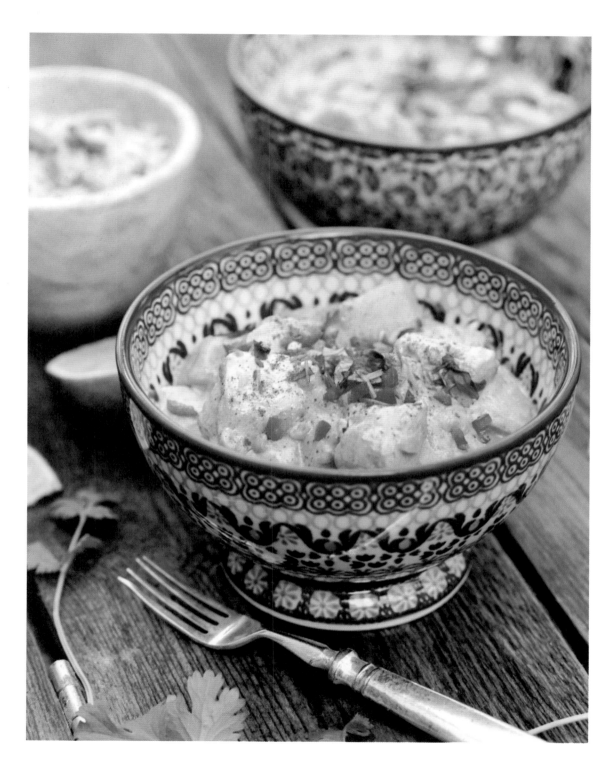

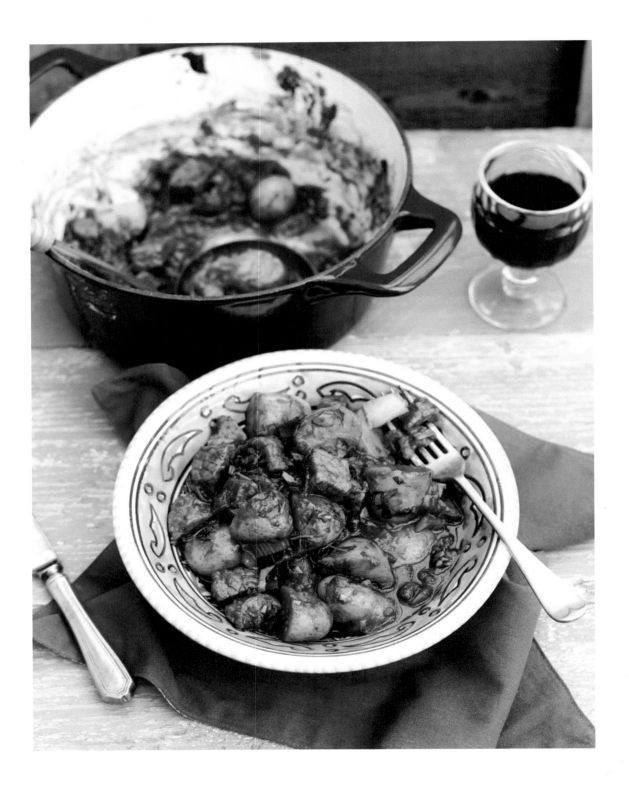

JOGGER'S BEEF STEW

LOG OUT.
SHUT DOWN.
GO RUN.

If you have 20 minutes to spare before you go out for a
run, then you can make this stew. It takes very little effort and
you don't have to be precise about the measurements either. I prepare this
and get it simmering before I go to the park for a one-hour running session. And I love
knowing that when I get back, there will be a healthy and tasty dinner waiting for me.

∘ ∘

SERVES 4

1 tsp olive oil

400g lean stewing beef, cut into 3cm pieces

1 onion, chopped

4 garlic cloves, crushed

4 celery sticks, chopped

1 tbsp dried mixed herbs

8 baby potatoes, halved

400g tin of chopped tomatoes

200ml vegetable stock

salt and pepper

chopped fresh oregano, to serve

Heat the olive oil in a large casserole over a
medium heat. Brown the beef in batches and set
aside on a plate. Reduce the heat and add the
onion and garlic. Cover and cook for 10 minutes,
stirring occasionally so that the onion and garlic
do not stick to the pot. Return the browned beef
to the pot. Add the celery, mixed herbs, potatoes,
tomatoes and stock. Stir well and bring to the
boil. Reduce to a low heat, cover and simmer
for 1½ hours.

Meanwhile, put on your runners and go for a jog!

When you are ready to serve, season to taste and
ladle the stew into warmed serving bowls.
Sprinkle over the oregano and serve.

BURRITO IN A BOWL

I don't eat a lot of takeaways but I never feel hard done by when I can make this kind of dinner. I love the flavours in this recipe and there's something great about eating it all together in a bowl. This recipe makes two big portions so you could reduce it – or try to keep some leftovers for lunch the next day.

○ ○

SERVES 2

3 tbsp olive oil

1 red onion, finely chopped

1 tsp cayenne pepper

1 tsp paprika

500g lean minced beef

125g brown rice

3 tbsp Greek or natural yoghurt

3 tbsp lime juice

3 tbsp tomato purée

60ml water

400g tin of kidney beans, drained and rinsed

½ iceberg lettuce, shredded

1 ripe avocado, peeled and sliced

100g Cheddar, grated

Heat the olive oil in a large pan over a medium heat. Add the red onion and cook for about 10 minutes, until softened. Add the cayenne pepper and paprika and cook for 1 minute. Stir in the mince and cook for about 10 minutes.

Meanwhile, cook the rice according to the instructions on the package. Mix the yoghurt and lime juice in a small bowl and set aside.

When the mince is cooked, stir in the tomato purée, water and kidney beans and heat through.

Divide the cooked rice between two serving bowls. Add a layer of iceberg lettuce to each one, followed by a layer of avocado slices and a layer of spicy mince. Sprinkle the Cheddar on top and finish with a dollop of the yoghurt mixture.

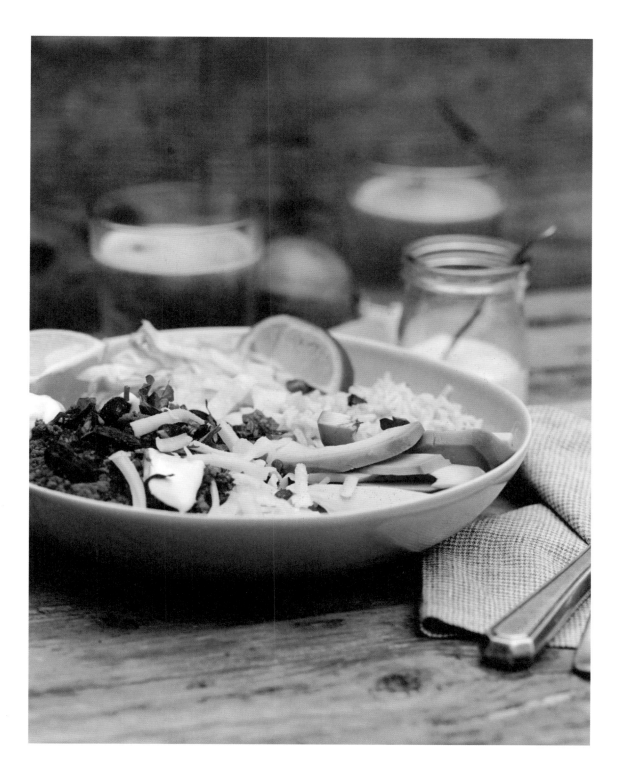

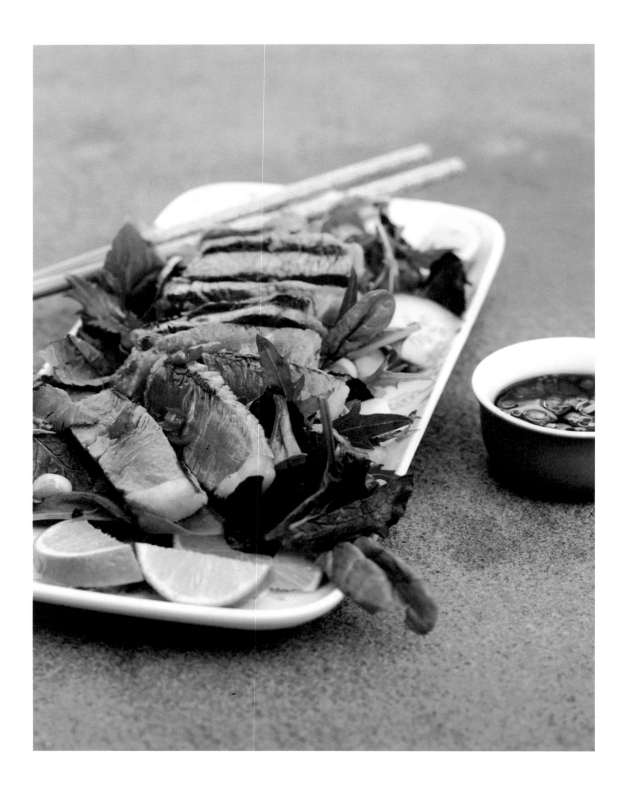

STEAK SALAD

I'm not really a salad girl at dinner time. If dinner is just a bowl of leaves, I won't be happy. This recipe does a lot for the reputation of salad. It's spicy and filling and so much more than the sum of its parts. If you want a bit more carbohydrate with it, you could serve a baked potato on the side.

○ ○ ○ ○ ○○

SERVES 2

For the salad

a handful of pine nuts
2 handfuls of mixed salad leaves
a handful of mint leaves, chopped
a handful of coriander leaves
a small bunch of scallions, trimmed and
    finely sliced
½ small cucumber, thinly sliced

For the dressing

2 garlic cloves, crushed
½ red chilli, finely chopped (more if you
    want a big kick)
2 tbsp lime juice
2 tbsp soy sauce
1 tbsp fish sauce
1 tsp agave
2 x 200 g rump or striploin steaks (about
    2cm thick), removed from the fridge
    30 minutes before cooking
olive oil
salt and pepper

Preheat the oven to 180°C/350°F/gas 4. Spread the pine nuts on a baking tin and bake for 5–10 minutes or until toasted, turning halfway through. Set aside to cool (but leave the oven on for the steaks).

Heat a grill pan or frying pan over a high heat. Rub both sides of each steak with a little olive oil. Season the steaks and place them in the pan. Cook for 2 minutes on each side. Lay the steaks in an ovenproof dish, cover with foil and place in the oven for 5–10 minutes. When the steaks are cooked to your liking, remove them from the oven and allow them to rest for 5 minutes.

Meanwhile, place all of the salad ingredients in a large serving bowl. Place all of the dressing ingredients in a jar with a lid and shake well to combine. Pour the dressing over the salad and toss well.

Use a sharp knife to cut the cooked steaks into thin strips. Arrange the steak strips on top of the salad and serve without delay.

STUFFED PEPPERS

I eat these stuffed peppers all the time – they're gorgeous. They're full of goodness and they make a complete meal when you serve them with rice, quinoa or couscous. Once they're in the oven, they pretty much take care of themselves.

○ ○ ○○

SERVES 1

2 tsp olive oil

2 shallots, finely chopped

2 garlic cloves, crushed

200g lean minced beef

2 tbsp soy sauce

2 tbsp tomato purée

200g tinned chopped tomatoes

1 pepper, halved lengthways and deseeded

2 tbsp grated Parmesan or 2 slices of mozzarella

a handful of mixed salad leaves

rice, quinoa or couscous, to serve

Preheat the oven to 180°C/350°F/gas 4.

Heat the olive oil in a large pan over a medium heat. Add the shallots and cook for about 10 minutes, until softened. Add the garlic and cook for 1 minute. Stir in the mince, soy sauce, tomato purée and chopped tomatoes and cook for 20 minutes, stirring occasionally.

Meanwhile, place the pepper halves on an ovenproof dish and bake for about 12 minutes, being careful not to burn them.

Carefully remove the peppers from the oven and spoon the cooked mince into them. Sprinkle over the Parmesan and return the peppers to the oven for 20 minutes.

Arrange the salad leaves on a serving plate alongside the stuffed peppers and serve with rice, quinoa or couscous.

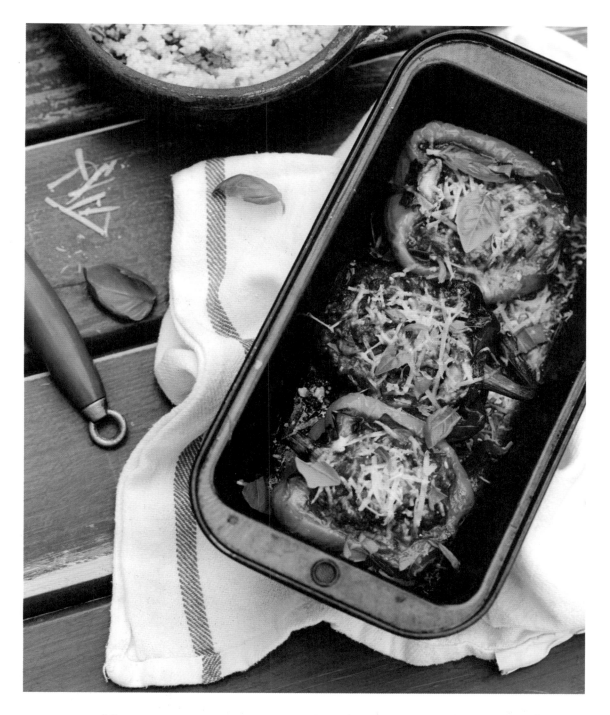

EAT LESS SUGAR: YOU'RE SWEET ENOUGH ALREADY.

This Shepherd's Pie also tastes great with a low-carbohydrate CAULIFLOWER MASH topping. Break two heads of cauliflower into florets. Boil in salted water until tender. Then drain, mash and stir in a little butter.

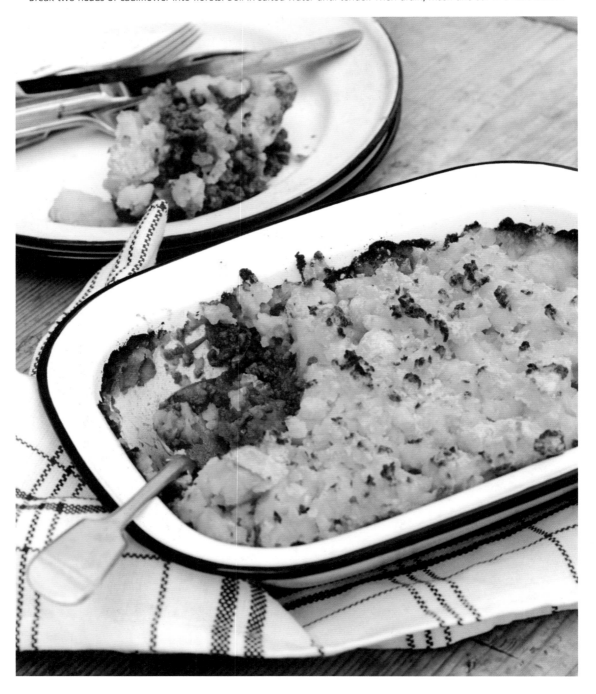

SHEPHERD'S PIE

If you're an Irish runner, you need to have this Shepherd's Pie in your repertoire! It is the ultimate antidote to running outside in the wind and rain. I'd also recommend that you buy a potato ricer to help you make recipes like this one. I use a potato ricer whenever I'm making mashed potatoes. Since the mash is so smooth and soft, there's no need to add too much butter. If the mash in this recipe is too indulgent for you, try a low-carbohydrate Cauliflower Mash instead.

○ ○ ○○ ○ ○○ ○ ○○ ○ ○○ ○ ○○ ○ ○○ ○ ○○ ○ ○○ ○ ○○ ○ ○○ ○ ○○ ○ ○○ ○ ○○ ○ ○○ ○ ○○ ○ ○○ ○ ○○ ○ ○○ ○ ○○

SERVES 2

1 tbsp olive oil

3 rashers, thinly sliced

2 onions, finely chopped

salt and pepper

1 tbsp dried herbs

2 garlic cloves, crushed

500g lean minced beef

300ml beef stock

100g peas

2 tbsp Worcestershire sauce

2 tbsp tomato purée

2 bay leaves

850g potatoes, peeled and quartered

40g butter

40g Cheddar, grated

100ml milk

Preheat the oven to 180°C/350°F/gas 4.

Heat the olive oil in a large pan over a medium heat. Add the rashers, onions, herbs and a pinch of salt. Cook for about 5 minutes, until softened. Add the garlic and cook for 2 minutes. Add the mince and cook for about 10 minutes, until browned. Stir in the beef stock, peas, Worcestershire sauce, tomato purée and bay leaves and bring to the boil. Reduce the heat, cover and simmer for about 5 minutes, stirring occasionally.

Meanwhile, make the mash. Boil the potatoes in salted water for 10–15 minutes, until tender. Drain, season and mash well. Stir in the butter, cheese and milk.

Place the cooked mince in a large ovenproof dish and top with the mash. Bake for 20 minutes. Divide the pie between warmed serving plates.

BEEF STIR-FRY

Stir-fries can be your saving grace during busy training periods. This one is quick to make and it has lots of lovely flavours and textures. It's my go-to stir-fry when I'm really busy.

○ ○ ○○ ○○ ○ ○○

SERVES 2

2 tbsp coconut oil

200g lean beef fillet, thinly sliced

1 carrot, peeled and finely sliced

a handful of baby corn, sliced lengthways

a handful of broccoli florets

a handful of sugar snap peas

a handful of shredded white cabbage

3 tbsp sweet chilli sauce

2 tbsp soy sauce

basmati rice, to serve

Heat the coconut oil in a large pan or wok over a medium-high heat. Add the beef and stir-fry for about 10 minutes, until browned all over. Remove the beef and juices and set aside.

Add all of the vegetables to the pan and stir-fry for about 5 minutes. Add the sweet chilli sauce and soy sauce and stir-fry for 2 minutes. Return the beef and juices to the pan, mix well and heat through. Divide the stir-fry between warmed serving plates and serve with basmati rice.

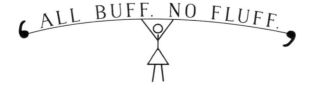

MOROCCAN MINCE & COUSCOUS

Tomato-based minced beef dinners can be stodgy and heavy – this Moroccan Mince is anything but. It has apricot, mint and lemon flavours so it's light and fresh. Served with the flavoured couscous, it makes a great meal.

○ ○ ○○ ○ ○○

SERVES 2

50g pine nuts

2 tbsp olive oil

2 onions, roughly chopped

1 tbsp ground cumin

2 tsp ground turmeric

1 tsp ground cinnamon

350g lean minced beef

600ml vegetable stock

100g dried apricots, quartered

280g couscous

4 tbsp chopped fresh mint

zest of 2 lemons

chilli oil, to serve

Preheat the oven to 180°C/350°F/gas 4. Spread the pine nuts on a baking tin and bake for 5–10 minutes or until toasted, turning halfway through. Set aside to cool.

Heat the olive oil in a large pan over a medium heat. Add the onion and cook for about 10 minutes, until softened. Stir in the spices and cook for 1 minute. Add the mince and cook for 5 minutes, stirring occasionally. Add the stock and apricots, stir well and bring to the boil. Reduce the heat and simmer, uncovered, for 20 minutes.

Meanwhile, cook the couscous according to the instructions on the package. Stir the mint and lemon zest into the cooked couscous.

Spoon the couscous into warmed serving bowls, making a well in the centre. Ladle the Moroccan Mince on top of the couscous and serve with a dash of chilli oil.

FIERY SPAGHETTI

I love making a big pot of this on a cold winter evening. Spicy pasta always feels comforting. You don't need any fancy ingredients for this recipe, so it makes for an easy and relaxed dinner when you've had a busy day.

∘ ∘

SERVES 2

2 tbsp olive oil
1 onion, finely chopped
3 garlic cloves, crushed
1 red chilli, finely chopped
400g tin of chopped tomatoes
300ml chicken stock
125ml white wine
500g lean minced beef
300g wholewheat or spelt spaghetti
salt and pepper
2 tbsp grated Parmesan, to garnish
a handful of basil leaves, to garnish

Heat a tablespoon of olive oil in a medium pan over a medium heat. Add the onion and cook for about 10 minutes, until softened. Add the garlic and chilli and cook for 2 minutes. Stir in the tomatoes, chicken stock and wine. Simmer, uncovered, for 30 minutes, stirring occasionally.

Heat a tablespoon of olive oil in a frying pan over a medium heat. Add the mince and cook for 20 minutes, stirring occasionally. When the mince is cooked through, transfer it to the pot with the tomato sauce and stir well. Simmer, uncovered, for 5 minutes.

Meanwhile, prepare the spaghetti according to the instructions on the package.

Divide the cooked spaghetti between warmed serving bowls. Season the spicy mince and ladle it over the spaghetti. Sprinkle over the Parmesan and basil and serve.

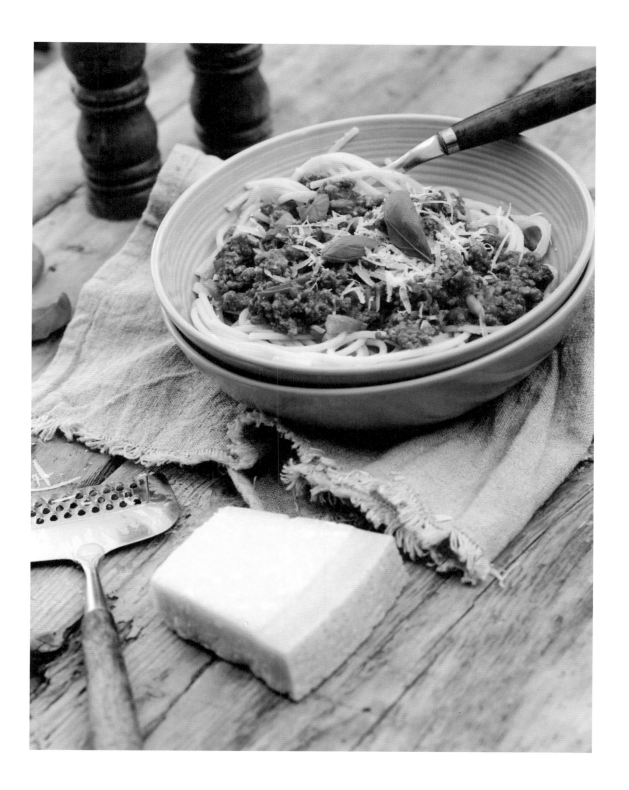

PLAYLIST

When I was a child, my parents used to say 'Run, Rabbit, Run!' before I started every race. I know – not the most technical advice. But whenever I was warming up for a big race, I had 'Run, Rabbit, Run' going around my head. There is something reassuring about keeping your thoughts simple, even when the stakes are high. I love music and I've always listened to music when warming up for training, weight lifting and big races. Lyrics in songs get me focused and relaxed all at the same time. Here is some of the music that might appear on my playlist.

- 'SURVIVOR' by Destiny's Child (I know this is such a girl anthem song but I love it. Don't judge!)
- 'NO GOOD (Start the Dance)' by The Prodigy (old-school classic)
- 'I'M STILL STANDING' by Elton John (this song makes me smile and run fast – win-win!)
- 'THIS IS WAR' by Thirty Seconds to Mars (great tune)
- 'CIRCUS' by Britney Spears
- 'YOU NEED ME, I DON'T NEED YOU' by Ed Sheeran
- 'IF I RULED THE WORLD' by Nas (feat. Lauryn Hill)
- 'ROYALS' by Lorde (great warm-down song)
- 'MEET ME ON THE EQUINOX' by Death Cab for Cutie
- 'THAT'S NOT MY NAME' by The Ting Tings (this is for the many, many people who insist that my name is Dervla – IT'S DERVAL!!!)
- COLLISION COURSE album by Jay-Z and Linkin Park
- THE HEIST album by Macklemore & Ryan Lewis

BAKED COD & LENTIL DAL

You don't need to buy a load of fancy ingredients for this Lentil Dal. It is no fuss and it tastes amazing with baked cod. It makes a quick nutritious dinner, even if you leave out the cod and just serve it with some brown rice. I make a big pot of this Lentil Dal once a week.

SERVES 2

1 tbsp coconut oil
1 onion, finely sliced
2 garlic cloves, crushed
½ red chilli, deseeded and finely chopped
a thumb-sized piece of ginger, peeled and grated
1 tsp ground coriander
½ tsp dried cumin
½ tsp medium curry powder
125g puy (dark green) lentils
1 tbsp tomato purée
400ml water
salt and pepper
2 x 180g cod fillets, skinned and pinboned
2 tbsp Greek or natural yoghurt, to garnish
chopped fresh coriander, to garnish

Preheat the oven to 180°C/350°F/gas 4.

Heat the coconut oil in a large pan over a medium heat. Add the onion and cook for about 10 minutes, until softened. Add the garlic, chilli, ginger and spices and cook for 1 minute, stirring all the time. Stir in the lentils, tomato purée and water and bring to the boil. Reduce the heat, cover and simmer for 35 minutes.

Meanwhile, season the cod fillets, wrap them in foil and place them on an ovenproof dish. Bake for about 25 minutes.

When the dal is cooked, check the seasoning and ladle it into warmed serving bowls. Place the cooked cod on top and garnish with the yoghurt and coriander.

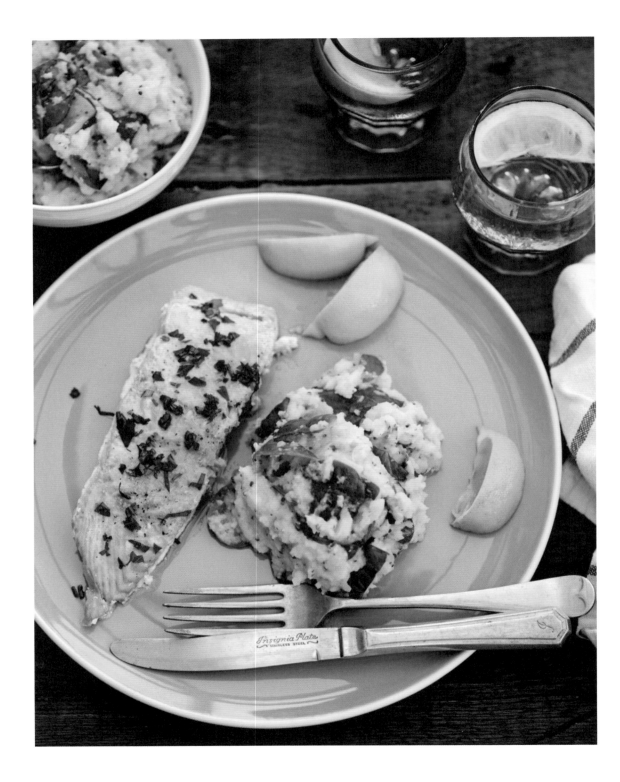

GRILLED SALMON WITH CELERIAC SPINACH MASH

This recipe title is a bit of a tongue-twister but I'm not kidding you: it's easier to make this recipe than it is to pronounce the title. We are so spoiled in Ireland to have such good-quality salmon available. It's delicious but it's also a brilliant protein source. I try to eat lots of salmon because of its amazing omega-3 benefits.

If you haven't cooked celeriac before, don't be put off by its ugly appearance. I have a vegetable equality policy and so should you.

SERVES 2

1 celeriac, peeled and cubed
100g baby spinach
2 x 100g salmon fillets, skinned and pinboned
2 tsp wholegrain mustard
1 tbsp olive oil
juice of ½ lemon
a pinch of pepper
a pinch of salt
2 tbsp Greek or natural yoghurt

Preheat the grill to medium and line a baking tin with foil.

Boil the celeriac in salted water for 15 minutes or until tender. Drain, then mash well in the saucepan. Once the mash is smooth, return the pan to a low heat. Stir in the spinach and cook, uncovered, or until the spinach has wilted.

Meanwhile, place the salmon fillets on the prepared tin. Mix the mustard, olive oil, lemon juice, pepper and salt in a small bowl. Lightly coat the salmon fillets with the mustard dressing, keeping some aside for later. Cook the salmon fillets under the grill for 10–15 minutes on each side, until golden and cooked through.

A few minutes before serving, add the yoghurt and one tablespoon of the mustard dressing to the celeriac and spinach mash. Stir well and season to taste. Divide the mash between warmed serving plates and arrange the salmon fillets on top. Drizzle over the remaining mustard dressing and serve.

BAKED TROUT WITH LIME & GARLIC BUTTER

It is worth making this recipe just for the lime and garlic butter, which goes really well with all sorts of fish. This recipe is a little indulgent but not too much work.

○ ○

SERVES 2
1 tbsp butter, softened
juice and zest of ½ lime
2 tbsp finely chopped fresh parsley
1 garlic clove, crushed
salt and pepper
2 x 100g trout steaks, pinboned
Sweet Potato Mash (p.122), to serve

Preheat the oven to 200°C/400°F/gas 6.

Combine the butter, lime zest, parsley and garlic in a small bowl. Season, mix well and set aside.

Place the trout steaks on a sheet of foil. Make 2–3 incisions in each steak and stuff the incisions with the herb butter. Squeeze a little lime juice over each steak and seal the foil. Place the steaks in an ovenproof dish and bake for 10 minutes. Then open the foil and bake uncovered for 10–15 minutes, until the fish is cooked and the skin is nice and crispy.

Place the cooked steaks on warmed serving plates and squeeze over a little lime juice. Serve with Sweet Potato Mash.

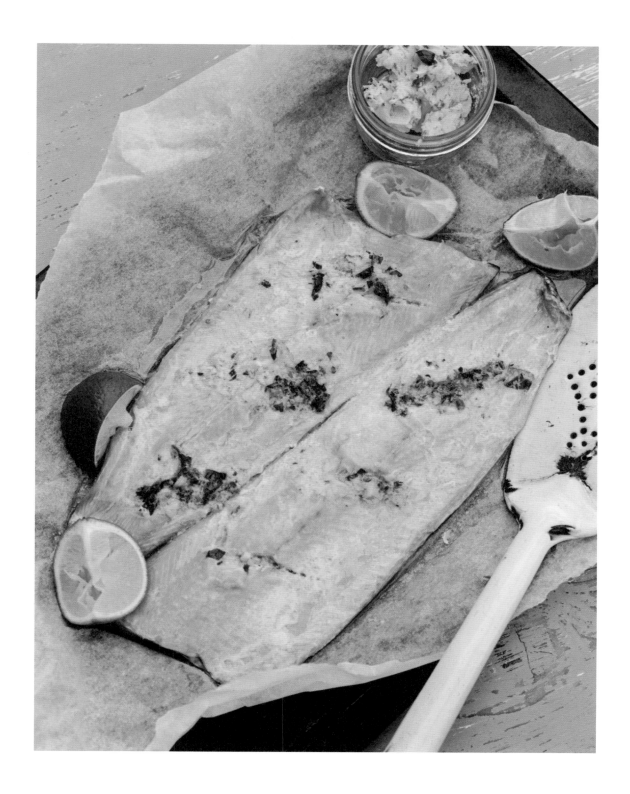

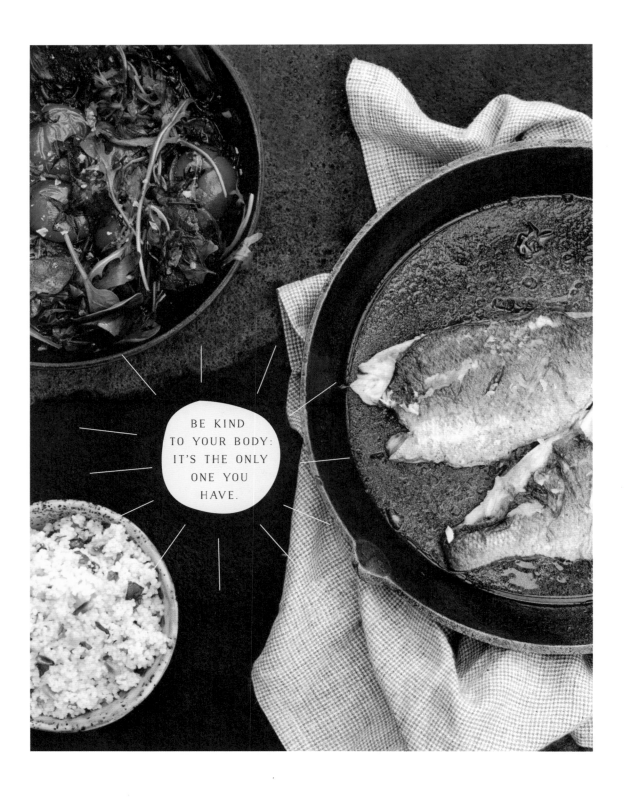

BE KIND
TO YOUR BODY:
IT'S THE ONLY
ONE YOU
HAVE.

SEA BASS WITH TOMATO & CHORIZO

This recipe sounds really cheffy but it's very quick and easy. It's a great one to make when you have friends over and you want a dinner that has nutritional value but also feels like special occasion food.

○ ○ ○○

SERVES 2

olive oil

12 cherry tomatoes, halved

6 wafer-thin slices of chorizo, halved

salt and pepper

170g couscous

2 x 100g sea bass fillets, skin lightly scored (turbot or brill also work well)

a handful of rocket

a handful of baby spinach

juice of 1 lemon

Heat a tablespoon of olive oil in a large pan over a medium heat. Add the tomatoes and chorizo. Season and cook for about 10 minutes, stirring occasionally.

Meanwhile, cook the couscous according to the instructions on the package.

Heat a tablespoon of olive oil in a large frying pan over a medium heat. Season the sea bass fillets and place them, skin-side down, in the pan. Cook for 1–2 minutes on each side, until the fish is cooked through and the skin is crispy.

Just before serving, add the rocket and spinach to the tomato mixture. Cook for about 30 seconds, stirring all the time.

Divide the couscous between warmed serving bowls and top with the cooked sea bass. Ladle the tomato sauce over, drizzle with lemon juice and serve.

BAKED HAKE & SMASHED SPUDS

I like to include fish in my diet whenever I get the opportunity. We are pretty spoiled to be living on an island – we should make the most of it. I try to eat fish two or three times a week. This baked hake is full of flavour and goes really well with the smashed spuds.

○ ○

SERVES 4

For the hake

4 x 100g hake fillets, skinned
    and pinboned
olive oil
salt and pepper
juice of 1 lime
a handful of chopped fresh
    chives

For the spuds

600g baby potatoes, unpeeled

For the salad

4 handfuls of mixed leaves
a handful of pumpkin seeds
a handful of Sweet & Sticky
    Pecans (p.166)
juice of 1 lime

Preheat the oven to 180°C/350°F/gas 4. Line a baking tin with foil.

Place the hake fillets on the prepared tin. Lightly coat them with olive oil and season generously. Drizzle over the lime juice and sprinkle over the chives. Cover the fillets with foil and set aside.

Boil the potatoes in salted water for 10–15 minutes, until tender. Drain well, then spread them out on a large roasting tin. Use the back of a fork or a rolling pin to smash the potatoes so that they are flattened and broken up (but not mashed). Season the smashed potatoes and give them a generous drizzle of olive oil.

Bake the hake and potatoes for 20–30 minutes, until piping hot and cooked through.

When you are ready to serve, place all of the salad ingredients in a large bowl. Drizzle over a little olive oil and toss well.

Divide the cooked hake between warmed serving plates and serve with the smashed potatoes and salad.

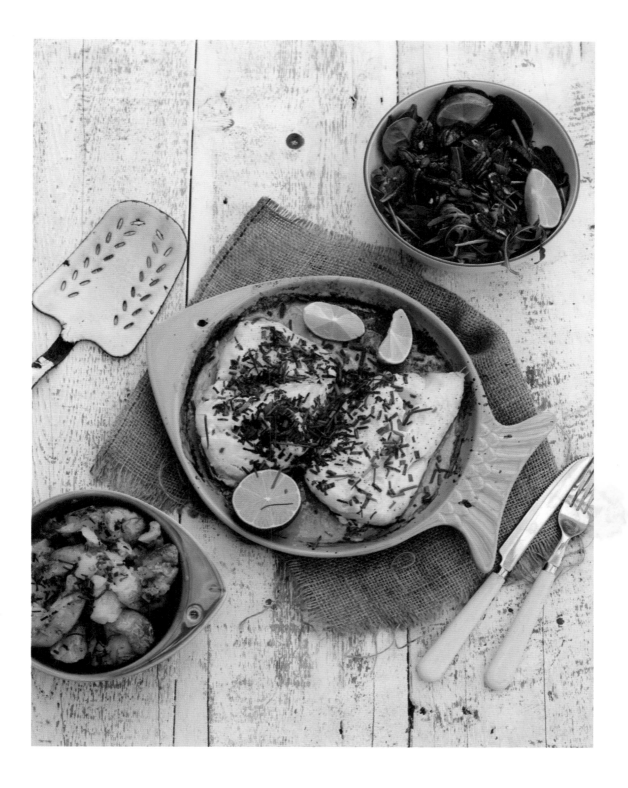

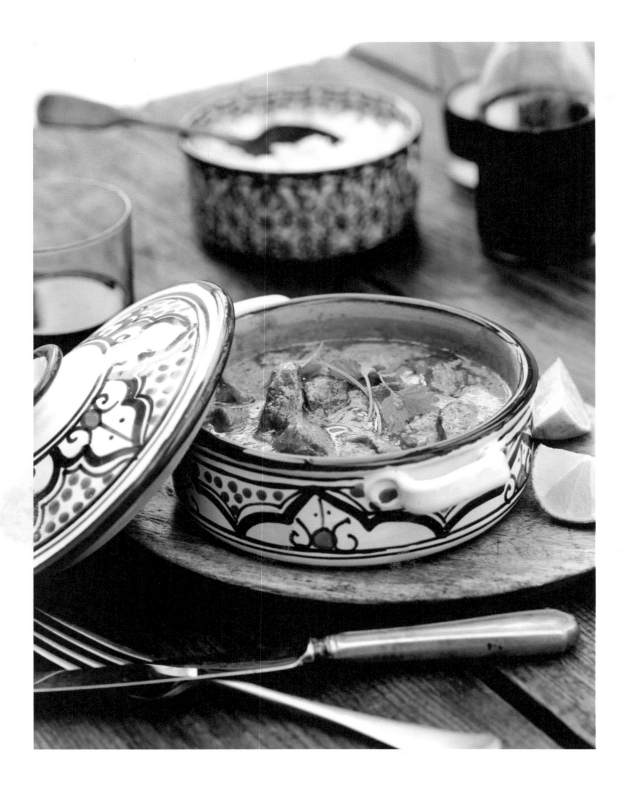

LAMB CURRY

This curry is easy to make – it just takes a bit of planning because you need to marinate the lamb first. I usually prepare the lamb and marinade and then head out for a training session. Two hours later the exercise is done, the lamb is tender and I can get cooking.

○ ○

SERVES 4

1 lime, zest and juice
3 garlic cloves, crushed
800g shoulder of lamb, trimmed and
    diced into 3cm pieces
3 tbsp coconut oil
1 onion, finely chopped
2 tsp curry powder
1 tsp cumin
400ml tin of coconut milk
2 tbsp tomato purée
1 tbsp hot pepper sauce or tabasco
2 tsp agave syrup
chopped fresh coriander, to garnish
brown rice or couscous, to serve

Mix the lime zest, juice and garlic in a large bowl. Add the lamb and use your hands to massage the marinade into the meat. Cover and leave to marinate in the fridge for 2 hours.

Heat the coconut oil in a large casserole over a medium heat. Add the onion and cook for about 5 minutes. Drain the lamb and discard the marinade. Cook the lamb in batches in the casserole, until browned on all sides. Stir in the curry powder and cumin and cook for 1 minute. Stir in the coconut milk, tomato purée, hot pepper sauce and agave syrup and cook for about 5 minutes. Reduce the heat, cover and simmer for 1½ hours. Stir occasionally and add a little water to the casserole if the curry seems dry.

Ladle the curry into warmed serving bowls and sprinkle over the coriander. Serve with brown rice or couscous.

CREAMY PISTACHIO PASTA

I first cooked a version of this in Dublin Cookery School under the guidance of cooking legend Lynda Booth. It's my twist on Carbonara. It's pure indulgence, with plenty of cream and Parmesan. I sometimes have this for a Meatless Monday dinner. It's an indulgence, though, so don't make it all the time!

° °

SERVES 2

1 tbsp olive oil

1 onion, finely chopped

4 tbsp crushed pistachios

½ red chilli, finely chopped

180ml cream

100g spelt pasta

2 tbsp Parmesan, grated

a handful of mint leaves, chopped

2 tbsp sunflower or pumpkin seeds

salt and pepper

Heat the olive oil in a large pan over a medium heat. Add the onion and cook for 5 minutes. Add the pistachios and chilli and cook for 5 minutes. Stir in the cream, reduce the heat and simmer for 5 minutes.

Meanwhile, cook the pasta according to the instructions on the package. Drain the pasta and tip it into the pan with the cream sauce. Add the Parmesan, mint and seeds and stir well to coat the pasta. Season to taste and divide the pasta between warmed serving bowls.

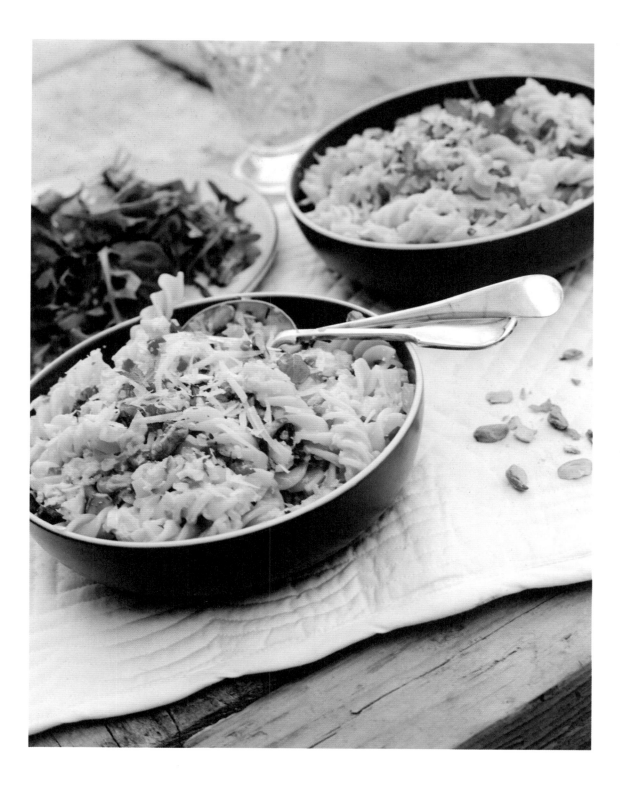

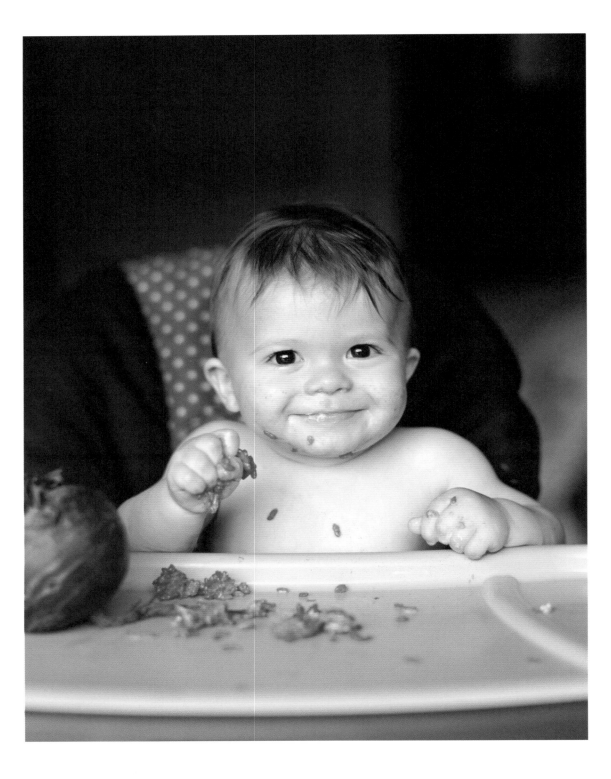

KEANE'S BEETROOT RISOTTO

This is my take on a *Bon Appétit* recipe I came across on www.epicurious.com. I first tested it in my friend Karen Shinkins's house in Atlanta with her baby – my godson, Keane – crawling around and watching every move I made in his kitchen. Little Keane was about a year old at the time and he loved the colour and the taste of the risotto. I was due to run a big track meet the next day, so a bright-pink dinner was actually a great distraction for me too.

° ○ ° ○

SERVES 2

50g butter

1 beetroot, peeled and grated

½ onion, finely chopped

1 garlic clove, crushed

130g risotto rice (pearl barley also works well but you need to parboil it for 20 minutes)

1 tbsp balsamic vinegar

300ml vegetable stock, simmering

salt

100g goat's cheese or feta

a large handful of spinach or rocket, to garnish

Melt the butter over a low heat in a large heavy-based saucepan. Add the beetroot and onion and cook for about 10 minutes, until softened. Stir in the garlic and rice and cook for 2–3 minutes. Stir the balsamic vinegar into the stock. Add the stock to the pan a ladleful at a time, stirring constantly, until each ladleful is absorbed. This will take about 30 minutes.

When the rice is creamy but firm to the bite, season with a pinch of salt. Spoon the risotto into warmed serving bowls. Crumble over the goat's cheese, garnish with the spinach and serve.

VEGETABLE TAGINE WITH MINTY COUSCOUS

I like to challenge myself to have the occasional Meatless Monday. This recipe is lovely for dinner and it tastes super the next day as well. There's a great mix of vegetables too, so it's packed full of vitamins and minerals. If you really can't resist having some meat, serve this with chicken.

SERVES 4

For the tagine

3 tbsp olive oil
1 large onion, finely chopped
1 tbsp ginger, finely chopped
1 garlic clove, crushed
2 tsp cinnamon
1 tsp cumin
1 aubergine, diced
1 carrot, peeled and diced
1 parsnip, peeled and diced
½ butternut squash, peeled, deseeded and diced
400g tin of chopped tomatoes
100g dried apricots, halved
zest of 1 lemon
300ml water
3 tbsp harissa
2 tbsp honey
2 tbsp tomato purée
salt and pepper

For the couscous

400g couscous
a handful of mint leaves, chopped
a handful of flaked almonds
2 tbsp olive oil

Heat the olive oil in a large pan over a medium heat. Add the onion and cook for 10 minutes, until softened. Add the ginger, garlic, cinnamon and cumin and cook for 2 minutes. Add the remainder of the ingredients for the tagine and stir well. Cover and simmer for 40 minutes.

Meanwhile, cook the couscous according to the instructions on the package. Stir the mint, almonds and olive oil into the cooked couscous.

Spoon the couscous into warmed serving bowls, making a well in the centre. Ladle the Vegetable Tagine on top of the couscous and serve.

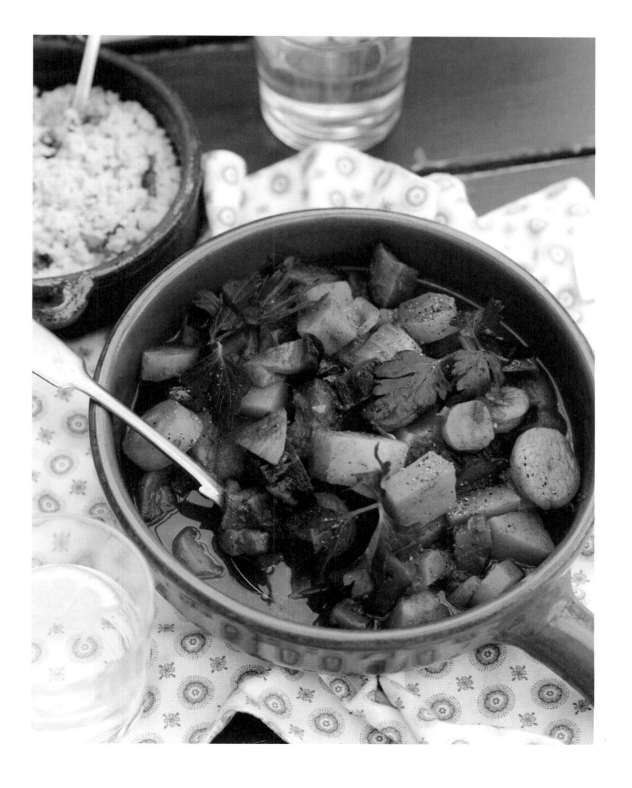

SIDES, SNACKS & DRINKS

CARROTS
& OATS

This is a lovely side. The oats make a nice crispy top on the carrots, and the butter is a little indulgent but totally worth it. I love any excuse to eat some nuts, so I've included almonds in this recipe.

SERVES 2

25g porridge oats
20g flaked almonds
3 carrots, peeled and sliced
2 tsp butter, melted

Preheat the oven to 180°C/350°F/gas 4.

Mix the oats and almonds in a small bowl and set aside.

Boil the carrots in lightly salted water for 5 minutes. Drain and place in an ovenproof dish. Pour over half the melted butter. Tip in the oats and almonds and spread them evenly over the carrots. Pour over the remaining melted butter.

Bake for 25 minutes, until the top is golden and crispy.

RED
CABBAGE
& APPLE

This is a yummy side for roast chicken and it's full of nutrition. It's also great with beef or fish.

SERVES 4

2 tbsp olive oil
1 onion, finely chopped
1 tsp fennel seeds
a pinch of salt
1 small head of red cabbage, finely sliced
2 eating apples, peeled, cored and chopped
60ml balsamic vinegar
50g walnuts, chopped

Heat the olive oil in a large heavy-based saucepan over a medium heat and add half of the onion. Stir in the fennel seeds and a pinch salt and cook for 1–2 minutes. Add the cabbage, apples and vinegar and cook for about 5 minutes, stirring well. Reduce the heat and cover. Cook over a low heat for 45 minutes to 1 hour, stirring occasionally.

Transfer the Red Cabbage & Apple to a warmed serving bowl, sprinkle over the walnuts and serve.

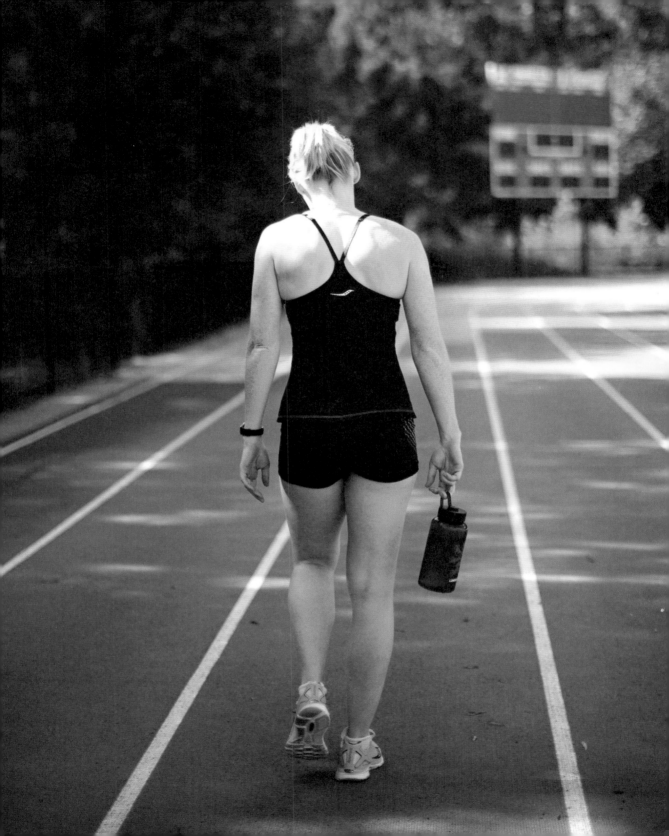

SWEET POTATO MASH

My relationship with sweet potatoes had a rocky beginning. I knew that sweet potatoes scored pretty well on the glycemic index but I also knew I loved the good old-fashioned Irish spud. I had to find a way for both kinds of potatoes to live in harmony in my diet. This recipe helped – and now I couldn't be without Sweet Potato Mash.

∘ ∘ ∘∘

SERVES 2

2 medium-sized sweet potatoes, scrubbed and left whole
3 tbsp orange juice
1 tbsp olive oil
¼ tsp garam masala
a pinch of salt

Cook the sweet potatoes in a microwave on a high setting for 3–4 minutes. (If you have the luxury of time, you could bake them in the oven for about 40 minutes either.)

Peel the cooked sweet potatoes and place them in a large mixing bowl with the rest of the ingredients. Mash to a smooth consistency and serve.

PITTA CHIPS

These Pitta Chips are a smart way to stay away from shop-bought tortilla chips or crisps. They're done in the oven and they are zero hassle. Make these and you'll get to enjoy your dips without eating any junk.

GOOD THINGS COME TO THOSE WHO ~~WAIT~~ WORK THEIR ASSES OFF AND NEVER GIVE UP.

○ ○ ○○ ○○ ○○ ○○ ○○ ○○ ○○ ○○ ○○ ○○ ○○ ○○ ○○ ○○ ○○ ○○

SERVES 2

2 wholemeal pitta breads
olive oil
salt and pepper
topping of your choice: chilli
    flakes, minced garlic, fresh
    herbs or grated Parmesan

Preheat the oven to 180°C/350°F/gas 4. Line a large baking tin with parchment paper.

Use a sharp knife to split the pittas in half and cut them into triangles about the size of a tortilla chip. Place the triangles on the prepared tin. Drizzle with olive oil, season and sprinkle over your chosen topping. (If using fresh herbs, sprinkle them over the pittas after baking.)

Bake the chips for 12–15 minutes, turning once.

Arrange the Pitta Chips on a serving platter alongside some dips or pesto.

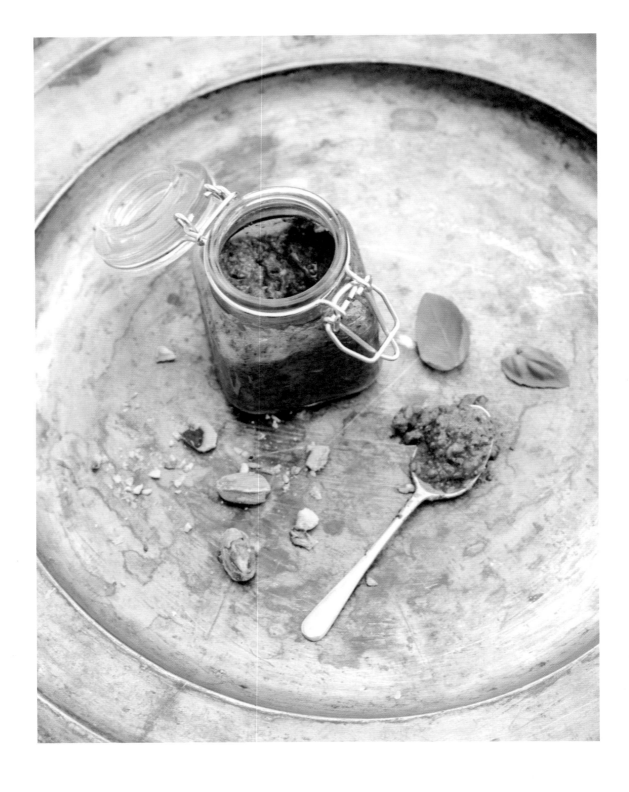

BASIL PESTO

Basil pesto is super-tasty and this is quite a healthy version. It can be enjoyed in sandwiches, as a dip or spread or as a sauce for pasta. You can use Parmesan, Pecorino or Grana Padano in this pesto – whatever's available. Remember that cheese goes a long way in pesto, so if you're looking for an even healthier version you could reduce the quantity of cheese by half.

This pesto will keep in a jam jar in the fridge for up to ten days. Just make sure you pour a thin film of olive oil over the top of the pesto before you put the lid on – this will seal in the flavour and keep the pesto from darkening.

o o o o o o o o o o o o o o o o o o o o o o o o o o o o o o o o o o o o o o

MAKES A SMALL JAR
1 whole fresh basil plant, leaves
    picked and washed but not dried
40g Parmesan, grated
40g shelled pistachios
2 garlic cloves, peeled
3 tbsp olive oil
2 tbsp water
½ tsp sea salt
a pinch of black pepper

Place all of the ingredients in a large mixing bowl and use a hand blender to blitz until the pesto reaches your desired consistency. (I like mine with a bit of texture.)

GUACAMOLE

Guacamole is a great dip for raw vegetables and it's good in salads too.

○ ○ ○○

MAKES A SMALL BOWL

1 ripe avocado, peeled and cubed

1 scallion, chopped

½ red chilli, deseeded and chopped

½ ripe tomato, chopped

salt and pepper

a squeeze of lime juice

Mash the avocado in a bowl. Stir in the rest of the ingredients and serve.

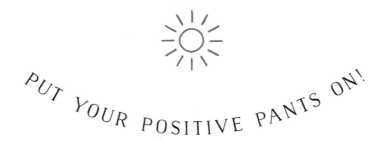

PUT YOUR POSITIVE PANTS ON!

ROAST PEPPER HUMMUS

Hummus is a great staple for nutritious snacking and it can really liven up sandwiches, crackers or even a slice of toast. This hummus is full of flavour because of the roasted peppers. It can be tricky to remove the skins from peppers after roasting them but I have a handy trick. Allow them to cool a little, put them in a plastic bag and then use your hands to rub the peppers through the bag. This hummus keeps in an airtight container in the fridge for up to 10 days.

MAKES A SMALL BOWL

4–6 peppers, halved and deseeded
2 tbsp olive oil
200g tinned chickpeas, rinsed
1 garlic clove
2 tbsp water
1 tbsp tahini paste
juice of ½ lemon
salt and pepper, to taste

Preheat the oven to 180°C/350°F/gas 4.

Spread the peppers on a large roasting tin and drizzle over the olive oil. Roast the peppers for 30 minutes. Remove the peppers from the oven and carefully take off the skins.

Place the peppers in a food processer, along with the remaining ingredients and blitz until you have a smooth hummus.

SMOKED MACKEREL PÂTÉ

Before my husband, Peter, sailed in two Olympic Games for Ireland, he took to the water for other reasons. He loves fishing. As a child, mackerel was his specialty catch.

MAKES A SMALL BOWL
100g smoked mackerel fillet, skin removed, flaked
100g cream cheese or cottage cheese
1 tbsp horseradish sauce
1 tbsp chopped chives
zest and juice of 1 lemon
salt and pepper

Place the mackerel, cream cheese and horseradish sauce in a large bowl and use a fork to mix well. Add the chives, lemon zest and juice and mix until thoroughly combined. Season to taste and serve.

TZATZIKI

This dip is summery and light and it goes perfectly with pitta chips. It's also great for barbecued meats such as chicken and lamb – and it's a much smarter nutritional choice than a lot of gloopy salad dressings.

MAKES A SMALL BOWL
½ cucumber, peeled, deseeded and finely chopped
1 garlic clove, crushed
200g Greek yoghurt
a handful of mint leaves, finely chopped
juice of ½ lemon
a pinch of salt and pepper

Place all of the ingredients in a large bowl and use a fork to mash to your desired consistency. Scrape the Tzatziki into a serving bowl.

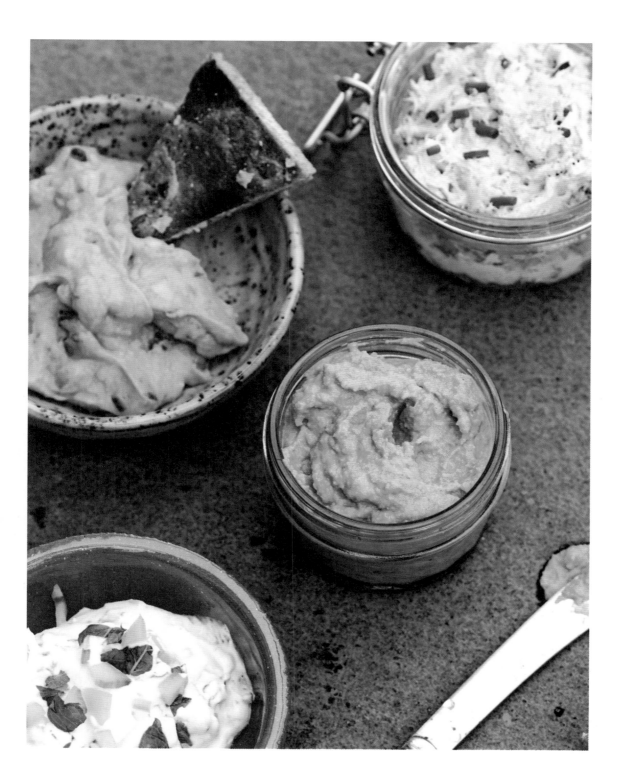

GRAB-AND-GO SNACKS

We all get busy and find ourselves in need of a snack. That's why this book is full of make-ahead snack ideas, so you never have to face the junk aisle if you don't want to. Of course, you won't always have the time to prepare snacks for the day ahead. If you're short on time but still want to eat well, try these zero-preparation snacks. Just grab – and go! • Dried fruit • Banana • Handful of mixed nuts • A few squares of dark chocolate • Apple pieces dipped in nut butter • Fruit smoothie • Vegetable juice • Handful of mixed berries • Pot of natural yoghurt • Rice cakes with nut butter

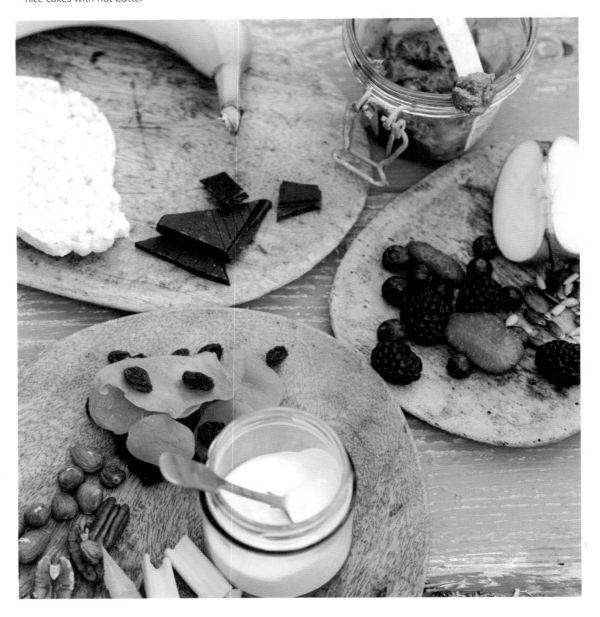

'

I LIKE TO EAT AND TRAIN,
NOT DIET AND EXERCISE.

'

JAM JAR DRESSINGS

It's a running joke in our house that I scrub and reuse any jam jar that comes through the door. I do this because I like to have loads of different options when it comes to salads, and jam jars are the handiest way to make and keep my own salad dressings. For each of the recipes below, just put the ingredients in a jam jar with a tightly-fitted lid and shake well to make your dressing.

○ ○ ○ ○

Asian-style

1 scallion, finely sliced
½ red chilli, finely chopped
6 tbsp olive oil
2 tbsp lime juice
2 tbsp soy sauce
1 tbsp agave syrup
1 tbsp chopped fresh coriander
salt and pepper, to taste

Parsley & Ginger

½-inch piece of ginger, grated
1 garlic clove, crushed
1 scallion, finely sliced
6 tbsp olive oil
2 tbsp white wine vinegar
1 tbsp chopped fresh parsley
salt and pepper, to taste

Agave & Mustard

6 tbsp olive oil
2 tbsp white wine vinegar
1 tbsp agave syrup
1 tbsp Dijon mustard
salt and pepper, to taste

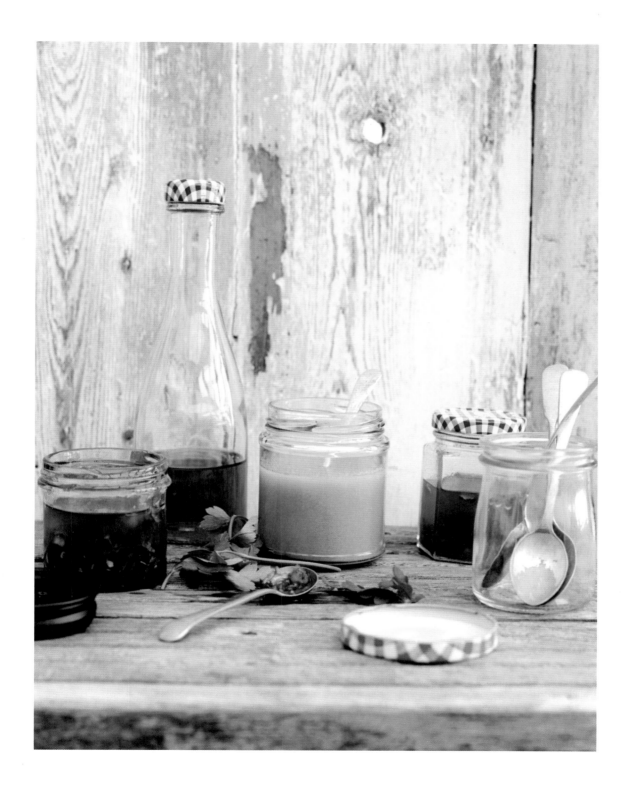

STOPWATCH
BROWN BREAD

A lot of people buy brown bread because they assume that it will take a long time and cost a lot of money to bake their own bread. Both assumptions are off the mark. Stopwatch Brown Bread costs very little to make and can be done from start to finish in under an hour.

∘ ∘

MAKES 1 LOAF

240g wholemeal flour
120g plain flour
1 tsp baking powder
½ tsp salt
350ml buttermilk
1 egg
1 tbsp agave syrup, plus extra for drizzling
30g pumpkin seeds
20g porridge oats

Preheat the oven to 180°C/350°F/gas 4 and lightly oil a 900g (2lb) loaf tin.

Sift the flours, baking powder and salt into a bowl.

Use a wooden spoon to mix the buttermilk, egg and agave in a large bowl. Pour the dry ingredients into the wet ingredients and mix until just combined.

Pour the dough into the prepared loaf tin. Top with a drizzle of agave and sprinke over the seeds and oats. Bake for 45 minutes until golden brown and well risen. Tip out onto a wire rack and leave to cool.

HAPPY, HEALTHY BREAD

My Happy, Healthy Bread is an adaptation of a recipe by cooking genius Sarah Britton. Sarah's website (www.mynewroots.org) is a great resource for healthy cooking. Every time I look at it I feel inspired.

In the past, I didn't eat a huge amount of bread. But once I started baking Happy, Healthy Bread I got hooked. I baked it regularly throughout the indoor season and I even brought some in a lunchbox on the plane to the European Indoor Championships. I ended up winning my fifth medal when I was there, so maybe the bread had something to do with it?

Happy, Healthy Bread is full of wholegrains, nuts and seeds. It is high in protein and fibre, and it contains psyllium seed husks. These husks suck up water and bind the bread together, so you don't need to use any flour. The bread is very easy to make, but you will need to let it sit for two hours before baking and you will also need a silicone loaf pan.

When I bake Happy, Healthy Bread I like to double the amount, slice the cooked loaves and freeze them. Then I can take slices out of the freezer as I need them. The bread tastes equally delicious whether it is baked fresh and allowed to cool or whether it is toasted. It is lovely with a little butter, jam or nut butter.

145g porridge oats

135g sunflower seeds

90g linseeds

65g brazil nuts, roughly chopped

4 tbsp psyllium seed husks

2 tbsp chia seeds

1 tsp fine sea salt (add an extra ½ tsp
if using coarse salt)

1 tbsp maple syrup (honey or agave
syrup also work well)

3 tbsp coconut oil, melted

350ml water

THINK POSITIVE,
EAT HEALTHY,
TRAIN OFTEN,
SLEEP WELL.

Mix all of the dry ingredients in a large bowl.

Whisk the maple syrup, coconut oil and water in a measuring jug. Pour this liquid into the dry ingredients and mix until combined. The dough should be very thick. If it becomes too thick to mix, add a few teaspoons of water until it is manageable.

Pour the dough into a silicone loaf pan and leave it to sit at room temperature for at least 2 hours. The dough is ready to be baked once it retains its shape when you pull the side of the loaf pan away from it.

Preheat the oven to 180°C/350°F/gas 4.

Place the loaf pan on the middle rack of the oven and bake for 20 minutes. Remove the bread from the loaf pan, place the bread upside down directly on the oven rack and bake for another 30–40 minutes. The bread is cooked once it sounds hollow when tapped.

Place the bread on a wire rack and leave it to cool fully before slicing. Store in an airtight container for up to five days or slice and freeze.

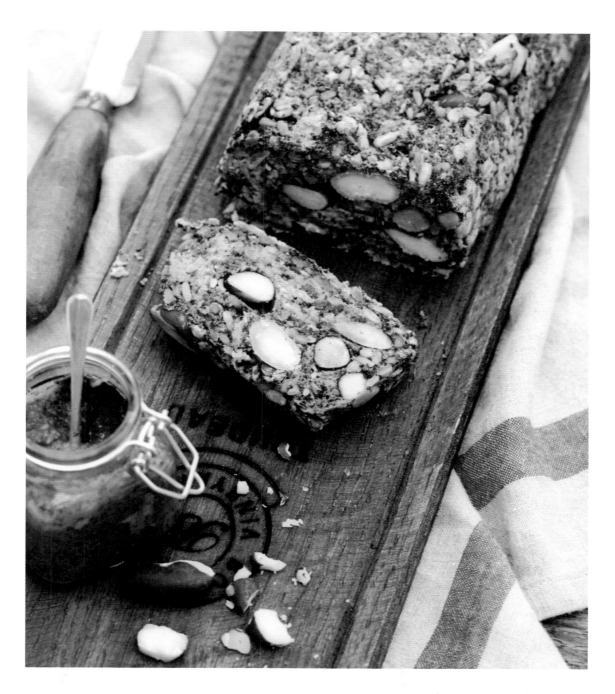

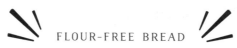

FLOUR-FREE BREAD

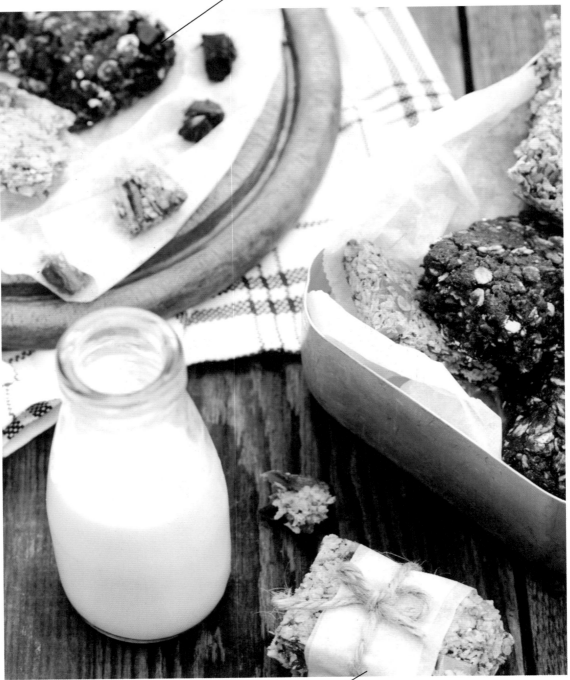

PETER'S FROZEN PROTEIN BARS

CHEWY GRANOLA BARS

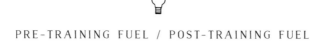

CHEWY GRANOLA BARS

It's easy to spend loads of money on seemingly healthy granola bars but it's a much better option to make these yourself. They're really handy to bring in your bag and eat at training, sitting in traffic or wherever else you find yourself.

○ ○ ○ ○ ○ ○ ○ ○ ○ ○ ○ ○ ○ ○ ○ ○ ○ ○ ○ ○ ○ ○ ○ ○ ○ ○ ○ ○ ○ ○ ○ ○ ○ ○ ○ ○ ○ ○ ○ ○

MAKES 12 BARS

120g jumbo porridge oats
50g desiccated coconut
50g pecan nuts, roughly chopped
1 tbsp chia seeds
3 tbsp water
3 tbsp honey
2 tbsp coconut oil
½ tsp vanilla extract
1 egg
2 medjool dates, chopped
30g dried mango, chopped
salt

Line a 33cm x 23cm (13 inch x 9 inch) metal baking tin with parchment paper so that the paper overlaps the sides. Preheat the oven to 150°C/300°F/gas 2.

Spread the oats, coconut and pecans on a baking tin and bake for about 10 minutes. Meanwhile, in a small bowl, mix the chia seeds and water to make a gel and set aside.

Melt the honey, coconut oil and vanilla extract in a large pan over a low heat. Remove from the heat and leave to cool slightly. Stir the chia gel into the honey mixture, one tablespoon at a time. (Ensure that each spoonful dissolves fully before adding the next.) Add the egg and stir until smooth. Stir in the dates, mango and a pinch of salt and mix well. Tip the toasted porridge mix into the pan and stir until combined.

Increase the oven to 180°C/350°F/gas 4. Scrape the granola mix into the prepared baking tin and spread out evenly, pressing down with the back of a spoon. Bake for 25–30 minutes until the top is golden brown and firm. Remove from the oven and leave to cool for 30 minutes. To remove from the tin, take hold of the parchment paper and simply lift out the granola slab. Cut the slab into bars and store them in an airtight container in the fridge.

PETER'S FROZEN PROTEIN BARS

This recipe makes some of the tastiest protein bars you'll ever have. Plus – there is no actual cooking in them. Win-win! Peter, my husband, makes these at least once a week and they are always gobbled up within a couple of days.

○ ○ ○○

MAKES 6 BIG BARS

300g chocolate protein powder (banana
   or vanilla flavours also work well)
160g jumbo porridge oats
70g sunflower seeds
50g dark chocolate (70% cocoa solids),
   chopped
30g ground almonds
1 banana, peeled and mashed
120ml water
3 tbsp coconut oil, melted
1 tsp vanilla extract

Line a 33cm x 23cm (13 inch x 9 inch) baking tin with parchment paper.

Place all of the ingredients in a large mixing bowl and use your hands to mash everything to a sticky consistency. This process will take a few minutes and the mixture must not be too wet, so do not panic and throw in more water. Simply keep working the mixture with your hands.

Scrape the mixture into the prepared tin and place in the freezer for at least 1 hour.

Remove the tin from the freezer and leave to stand for about 30 minutes. Cut the slab into bars and carefully remove from the tin. Store the bars in airtight plastic bags in the freezer. Take them out as needed – just give them a few minutes to defrost before eating.

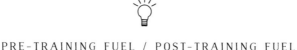

CHOCOLATE PROTEIN BARS

One of my major healthy habits is preparing in bulk the foods that are good for me and keeping them in the fridge until I need them. Quinoa is such a healthy food that I'm always looking for ways to incorporate it into my diet. I cook quinoa in big batches so that I can let it cool down and store it in the fridge until I need it. This recipe uses cooked quinoa along with loads of other nutritious and tasty ingredients.

MAKES 6 BIG BARS

For the bars

180g cooked quinoa
100g ground almonds
50g medjool dates, chopped
1 egg
4 tbsp honey
2 tbsp cocoa powder
2 scoops of vanilla protein powder
1 tsp ground cinnamon
1 tsp vanilla extract
½ tsp salt

For the topping

50g dark chocolate (70% cocoa
  solids), chopped
50g desiccated coconut

Line a 33cm x 23cm (13 inch x 9 inch) metal baking tin with parchment paper so that the paper overlaps the sides. Preheat the oven to 180°C/350°F/gas 4.

Place all of the ingredients for the bars in a large bowl and mix well. Scrape the mixture into the prepared baking tin and spread out evenly, pressing down with the back of a spoon to make the surface as even as possible.

Bake for 25–30 minutes until the top is golden brown and feels firm to the touch. Remove from the oven and leave to cool for at least 30 minutes. To remove from the tin, take hold of the parchment paper and simply lift out the slab. Cut the slab into bars.

Melt the chocolate in a heatproof bowl over a pan of simmering water. Partially dip each protein bar into the melted chocolate and sprinkle over some desiccated coconut. Leave the bars to rest on a wire rack for a few minutes. Once the chocolate has set, store the bars in airtight containers in the fridge for up to a week.

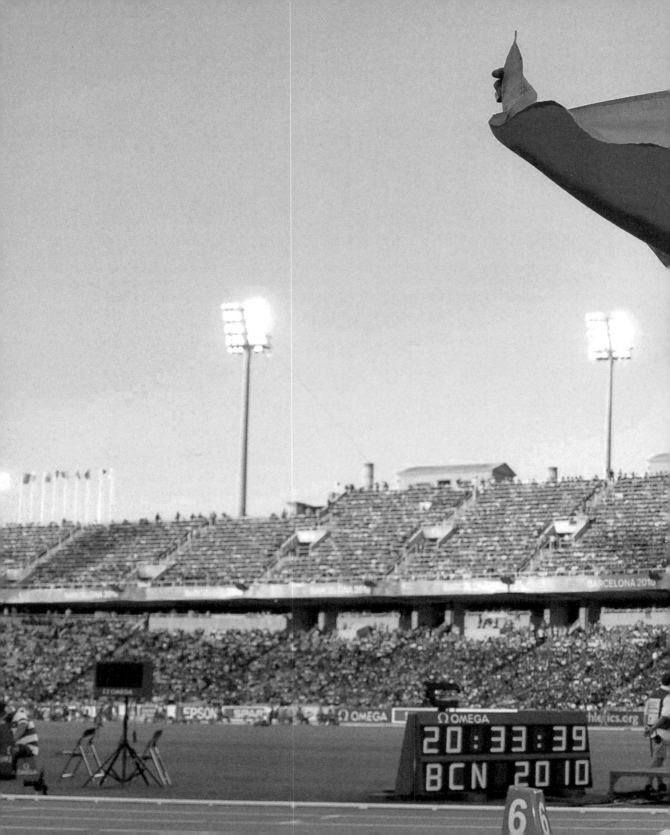

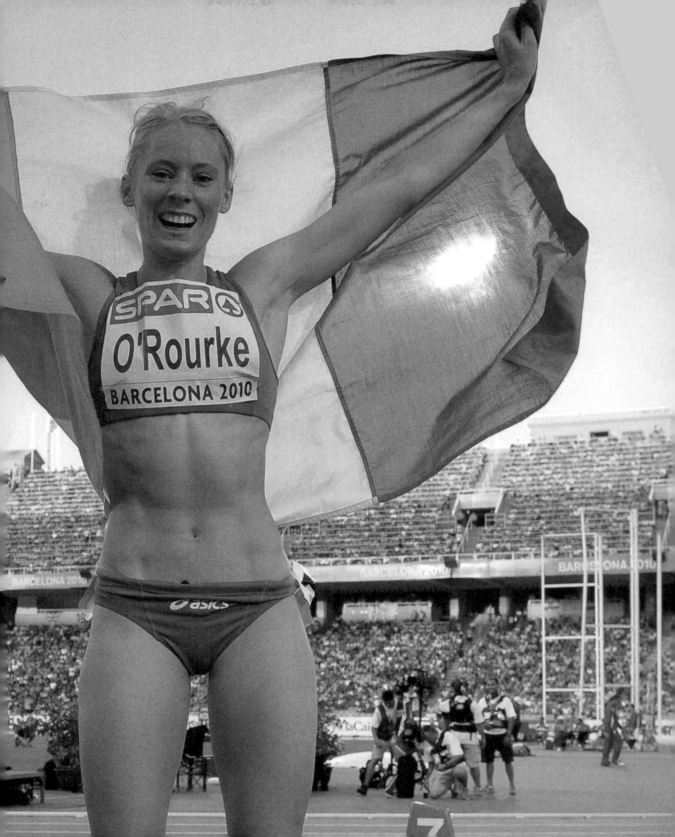

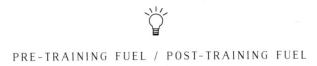

PEANUT & BANANA BOOSTERS

These no-bake bars are full of goodness and they give you a real boost because they
pack a bit of protein. They are really tasty and are no hassle to make.
I always have a batch of these in the freezer.

MAKES 6 BIG BARS

2 bananas, peeled

125g peanut butter

80g porridge oats

4 scoops of vanilla protein powder

2 tbsp chia seeds

a pinch of salt

Line a 33cm x 23cm (13 inch x 9 inch) baking
tin with parchment paper.

Place the bananas in a large mixing bowl, add
60ml water and mash until combined. Add the
rest of the ingredients. Mix well with a spatula,
ensuring that the peanut butter is thoroughly
combined. Scrape the mixture into the prepared
tin and place in the freezer for at least 1 hour.

Remove the tin from the freezer and leave to
stand for about 30 minutes. Cut the slab into
bars and carefully remove from the tin. Store
the bars in airtight plastic bags in the freezer.
Take them out as needed – just give them a few
minutes to defrost before eating.

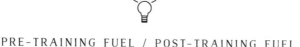

GREAT BALLS OF POWER

Goodness, gracious, Great Balls of Power! These little balls are like protein bombs.
They are a brilliant snack to have after a weights session. I always have a batch of them
in the fridge so that I can take a few with me when I'm on my way out to the gym.
They will keep in an airtight container in the fridge for up to two weeks but
I prefer to eat them within a few days.

MAKES 8–10 BALLS

8 tbsp crunchy peanut butter or almond butter
4 scoops of vanilla protein powder
4 tbsp agave syrup, honey or maple syrup
4 tbsp desiccated coconut
4 tbsp water
3 tbsp ground linseed
1 tsp vanilla extract

Place all of the ingredients in a large bowl and use your hands to mix it into a dough. Add a few drops of water if the mixture seems too dry. Use your hands to shape the dough into balls roughly the size of golf balls.

Place the balls in an airtight container and store overnight in the fridge. By morning, your Great Balls of Power will be ready to go.

TRAVEL TIME

I fly all the time. I take up to thirty return flights some years and I believe that flying well is a skill that improves with practice. If you see a flyer who is really well prepared and completely at ease, even on a long-haul flight, it is because they've had a bit of practice.

People fly for different reasons. I am in the business of running fast, so I fly to and from races – sometimes on the day of the race itself. I fly to training camps so that I can get sun on my back and speed in my legs. Over the years, I have become really organised with my own food when it comes to travelling. The idea of eating prepacked, barely edible plane food is not something that appeals to me.

Coming up to the World Championships in Daegu, I was dreading the flight. My coach Sean told me to pack all my own food. He said that from my door in Ireland to the door in South Korea, I was only to eat food that I had prepared myself. Off I went with my carry-on bag stuffed full of homemade snacks and mini-meals. When I arrived in South Korea I felt far better than after previous long-haul flights. I was well and truly ready to start training the next day.

And a few years back, I was on a flight to Atlanta for a training camp when I noticed one of the flight attendants smiling at me. When she passed down the aisle, she leaned in and said: 'The healthiest way to travel is to bring your own food with you. I've been doing that myself for years. Well done, Derval.' I can't tell you how proud me and my lunchbox were!

Pack FOODS THAT
HOLD their TEXTURE
and don't get excessively
mushy. I know from
experience that apples travel
better than oranges.

STAY HYDRATED while you travel.
Obviously, you can't bring homemade
drinks through airport security. My way
around this is to bring a water bottle with
a few lemon and ginger slices in it, and then
to fill up the water bottle once I've gone
through security. And I always find that
flight attendants are happy to fill up the
water bottle for you again when
you're on the flight.

If you want to pack
some dips and vegetables,
THINK ABOUT THE
CONSISTENCY first. Carrot
sticks and hummus usually travel
well. Just make sure the hummus
is in a see-through container
so that you can get it
through security.

SOME TIPS FOR TRAVELLING WITH FOOD.

Bring FOODS THAT
WILL LAST outside
the fridge for a few hours.
My Go Bananas! (p.16)
recipe is a very smart
choice.

AVOID PLANE
FOOD or eat just a
little bit of it. Most
of it is full of salt
and sugar.

AVOID COFFEE AND
ALCOHOL in airports and on
planes. These drinks do nothing
for your hydration: they just
make your jet-lag feel worse
in the end.

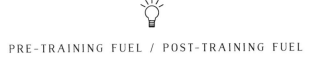

SUPER SNACKS

I always have a batch of these Super Snacks on the go. They're easy to make and they're a perfect post-training snack or healthy addition to an afternoon cup of tea. They will keep in an airtight container in the fridge for up to two weeks.

○ ○

MAKES 15 BALLS

75g desiccated coconut for the coating,
   plus 50g for the filling
225g dates
225g figs
150g flaked almonds
50g desiccated coconut
100ml water

Spread 75g desiccated coconut on a plate and set aside.

Place the dates, figs, almonds and 50g desiccated coconut in a food processor and blitz until combined. Add the water and blitz to form a sticky dough. Use your hands to shape the dough into balls roughly the size of golf balls. Then roll each ball in the desiccated coconut until coated. Your Super Snacks are ready to eat straight away.

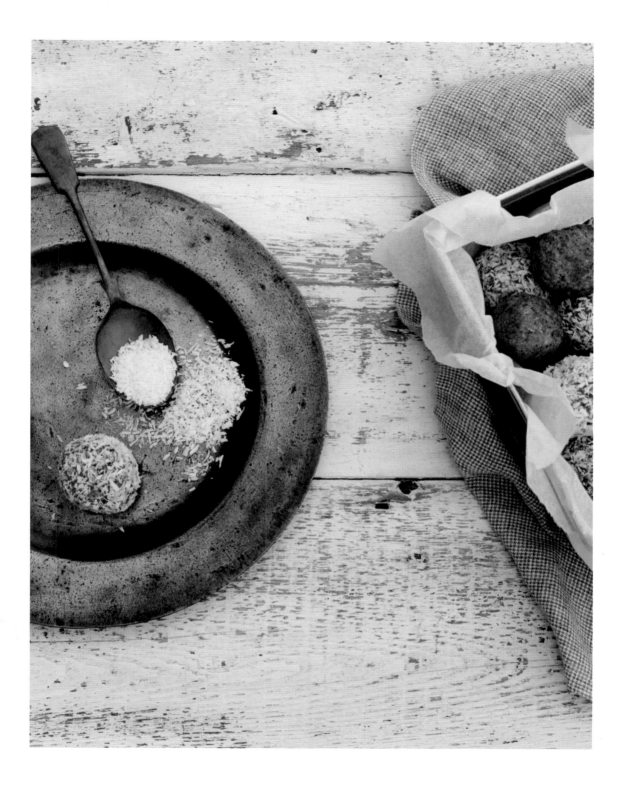

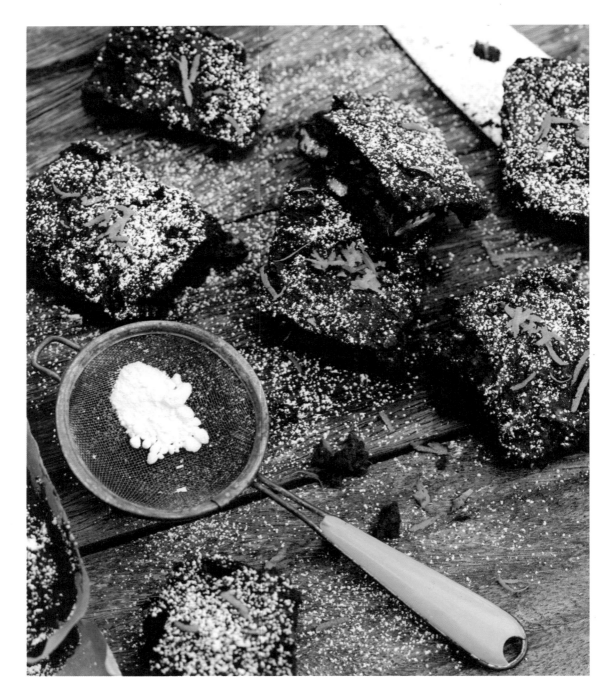

66 ALL YOU NEED IS LOVE (BUT A LITTLE CHOCOLATE NOW AND THEN DOESN'T HURT). 99

DARK CHOCOLATE & ORANGE ZEST BROWNIES

The primary ingredient in these brownies is actually sweet potato. I know that sounds weird but, believe it or not, these brownies taste amazing! It is absolutely worth the effort to make them. Just try not to scoff them all at once.

° °°

MAKES 6 BIG BROWNIES (OR 12 MINI)

400g sweet potato, peeled and cubed

100g dark chocolate (70% cocoa solids), chopped

½ tsp coconut oil

50g jumbo porridge oats

50g pecan nuts, chopped

1 tbsp cocoa powder

1 scoop of vanilla protein powder

½ tsp baking powder

½ tsp cinnamon

½ tsp salt

zest of 1 orange

3 egg whites

1 tsp agave syrup

Preheat the oven to 180°C/350°F/gas 4. Grease an 18cm (7 inch) square tin and line it with parchment paper.

Boil the sweet potato in salted water for 12 minutes or until tender. Drain, mash and set aside.

Meanwhile, melt the chocolate and coconut oil in a heatproof bowl over a pan of simmering water and set aside to cool slightly.

Mix the oats, pecans, cocoa powder, vanilla protein powder, baking powder, cinnamon, salt and orange zest in a bowl. Add the mashed sweet potatoes and stir well. Add the egg whites, agave and melted chocolate and stir until combined.

Pour the mixture into the prepared tin and bake for about 30 minutes, until firm in the centre and a skewer inserted comes out clean. Cut the slab into slices in the tin, then carefully remove the brownies to cool on a wire rack.

BANANA PROTEIN SMOOTHIES

Smoothies are a super-easy way to get something substantial into you. They are a smart nutritional choice and it's no big deal to make them. I keep stashes of frozen berries in my freezer so that I can make smoothies without any hassle. And because I include the protein powder, I feel like I'm getting a complete meal in a jiffy.

o o o o o o o o o o o o o o o o o o o o o o o o o o o o o o o o o o o o o o o o o o o o o o o o o o

Almond & Vanilla

SERVES 2

1 banana, peeled
1 tbsp almond butter or another
nut butter of your choice
1 scoop of vanilla protein
powder
200ml milk or rice milk

Place the banana in a blender
with the almond butter, vanilla
protein powder and milk and
blend until smooth and creamy.

Pour into a tall glass and serve.

Blueberry & Vanilla

SERVES 2

2 bananas, peeled
a large handful of blueberries
1 scoop of vanilla or banana
protein powder
300ml milk or rice milk
2 tbsp Greek or natural yoghurt
1 tbsp ground linseed

Place the bananas in a blender
with the blueberries, vanilla
protein powder, milk, yoghurt
and linseed and blend until
smooth and creamy.

Pour into a tall glass and serve.

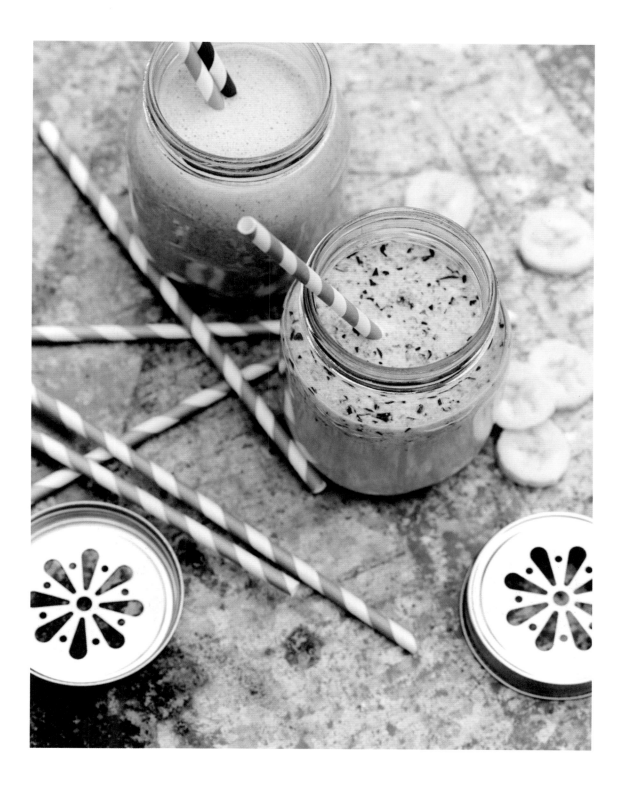

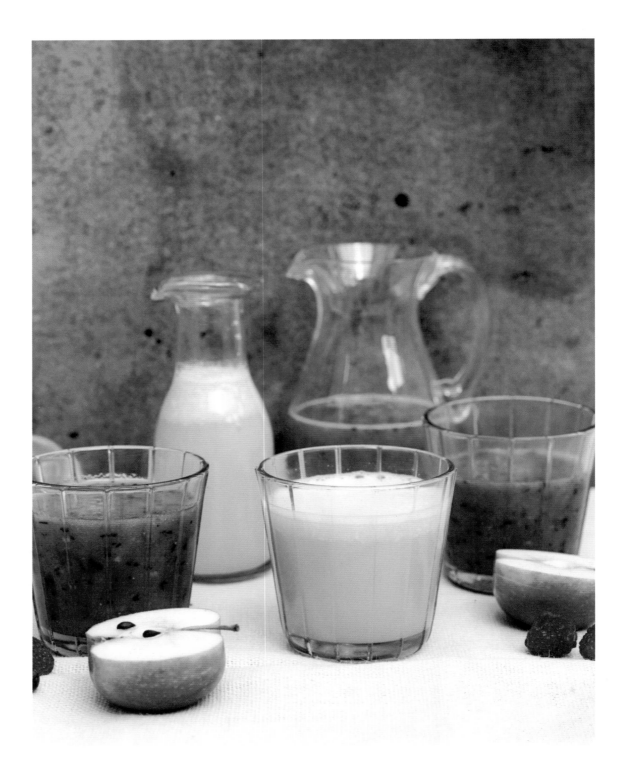

JUICES

My sister, Clodagh, is an expert when it comes to juices and smoothies! Whenever she comes to stay with me the first thing she does in the morning is make a fresh juice. She gave me the two recipes below. The Mango & Berry Juice is bursting with antioxidants, which are thought to promote anti-aging processes in the body. The Apple & Ginger Juice has anti-inflammatory properties and I believe it reduces stress on my muscles and joints after bouts of heavy training.

Ideally, you should use a juicer for these recipes. Juicers are troublesome to clean but they do allow you to make big batches of juice. Sometimes I use a regular blender to make juices. Whatever equipment you use, store homemade juices in airtight glass containers in the fridge. Drink homemade juices the same day you make them so that you maximise their nutritional benefits.

Mango & Berry

MAKES A JUG

2 mangos, peeled, stoned and roughly chopped
150g blueberries
150g strawberries
60ml water (plus extra, if you like a thinner juice)

Pass all of the fruit through a juicer. Stir in the water. Pour the juice into tall glasses and serve at once. Otherwise, store the juice in an airtight glass container in the fridge.

Apple & Ginger

MAKES A JUG

10–12 apples
a thumb-sized piece of fresh ginger, peeled

Pass the apples and ginger through a juicer. Pour the juice into tall glasses and serve at once. Otherwise, store the juice in an airtight glass container in the fridge. For an added health kick, add the juice of 1 beetroot.

SPRINTER SPRITZERS

In terms of hydration, I prefer to keep things as pure as possible. Plain water is a bit boring for me, though: I never want to drink a whole lot of it. I add different flavours to my water so that I can stay happy and hydrated. As a speed and power athlete, I don't have to worry quite as much as endurance athletes when it comes to hydration during training. My advice on sports and energy drinks is to read the label and choose the best drink for your needs. Be wary of the sugar and caffeine content in some products. If you are preparing for a big race – a 5km, 10km or marathon – practise your hydration during training to make sure that you get things right on the big day. After months of hard training, the last thing you'll want is to hit a wall because of dehydration. And even if you're not an athlete, it's a good idea to drink plenty of water. Use these Sprinter Spritzer recipes to dress up your water and you're bound to drink more of it.

○ ○

Lemony Goodness

I love my coffee first thing in the morning but sometimes I like to give myself a break with some hot water and lemon instead. It benefits digestion, boosts the immune system and has alkalising properties. Besides all that, it's such a refreshing way to kickstart the day.

500ml water, boiled and cooled
juice of ½ lemon

Vitamin C Boost

This flavoured water gives you a boost of Vitamin C, which is bound to put a spring in your step.

500ml water, boiled and cooled
½ lemon, sliced
½ lime, sliced
½ orange, sliced

Minty Lime

I grow mint because I never want to be without it. Mint is such a nice and versatile flavour and there's something soothing about it. If I'm nervous about something – a big training session or a race – I reach for a glass of Minty Lime.

500ml water, boiled and cooled
juice of ½ lime
a few mint leaves, torn

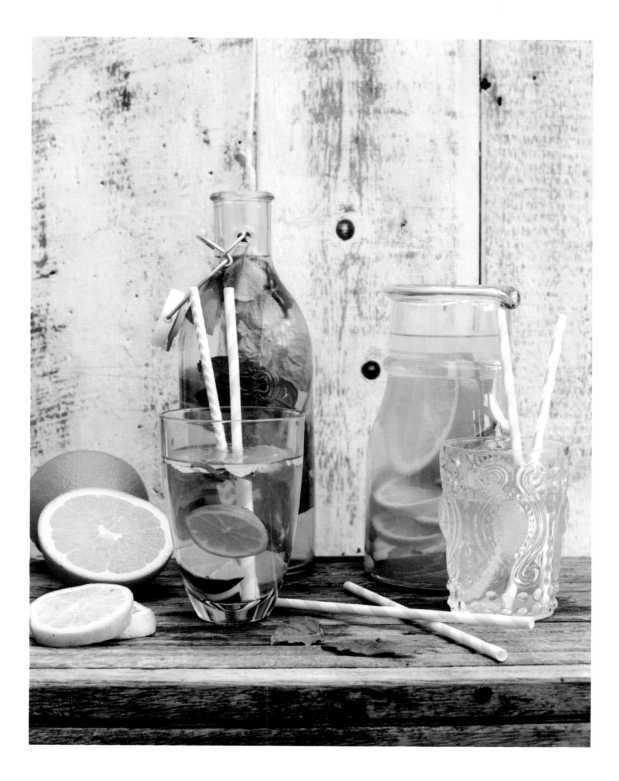

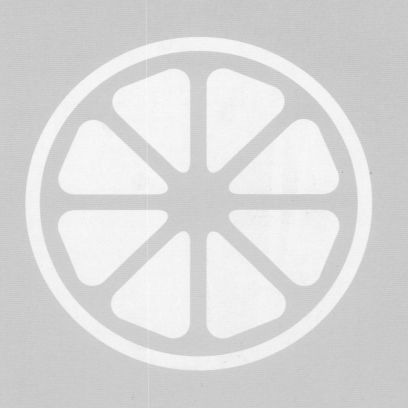

GINGERY LEMONY REMEDY

In our house, whenever Peter or myself feel sick we make the Gingery Lemony Remedy – or as we sometimes like to call it 'The Sick Drink'. When it looks like the sniffles are starting, we get sipping this stuff and we often find that we don't get any worse. So maybe the Gingery Lemony Remedy is the best medicine around?

MAKES ENOUGH FOR SEVERAL DAYS
a large chunk of ginger, grated
juice of 3 lemons
honey, as needed
boiled water, as needed

Mix the ginger and lemon juice in a small airtight container. This is the base for the Gingery Lemony Remedy and it must be stored in the fridge.

When you are ready to have a drink, mix 2–3 tablespoons of the base with 1 tablespoon of honey in a pint of boiled water. You should feel better in no time.

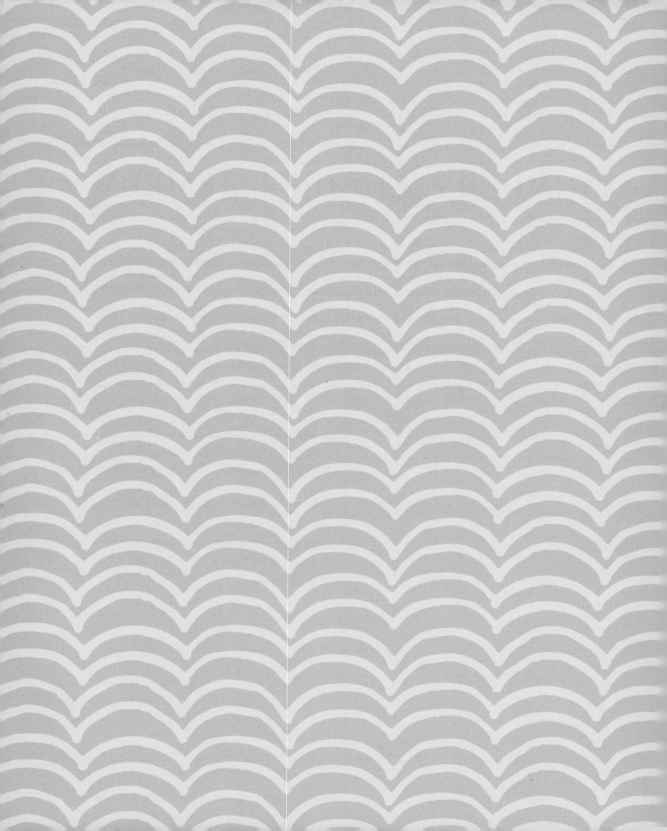

TREATS

DARK CHOCOLATE BANANA BREAD

What sets this bread apart is that it is made from a mix of different flours. Gram flour (also known as chickpea flour) is a great alternative to wheat flour. This banana bread is very easy to make and it comes out of the oven looking beautifully golden-brown. I love having a slice of this stashed away in my bag for a post-training-session treat.

MAKES 1 LOAF

2 ripe bananas, peeled
1 egg
40g maple syrup
3 tbsp coconut oil, melted
1 tsp vanilla extract
100g plain flour
50g gram flour
50g wholemeal flour
½ tsp baking powder
25g dark chocolate (70% cocoa solids), chopped

Preheat the oven to 180°C/350°F/gas 4. Grease a 900g (2lb) loaf tin and line it with parchment paper.

Use a fork to lightly mash the bananas in a mixing bowl and set aside.

Whisk the egg, maple syrup, coconut oil and vanilla extract in a large bowl with an electric beater until smooth. Sift the flours and baking powder into the bowl and mix until just incorporated. Stir in the banana and chocolate and pour the cake batter into the prepared loaf tin.

Bake for 30 minutes or until a skewer inserted comes out clean. Set aside to cool for 10 minutes, then remove from the tin and leave to cool on a wire rack.

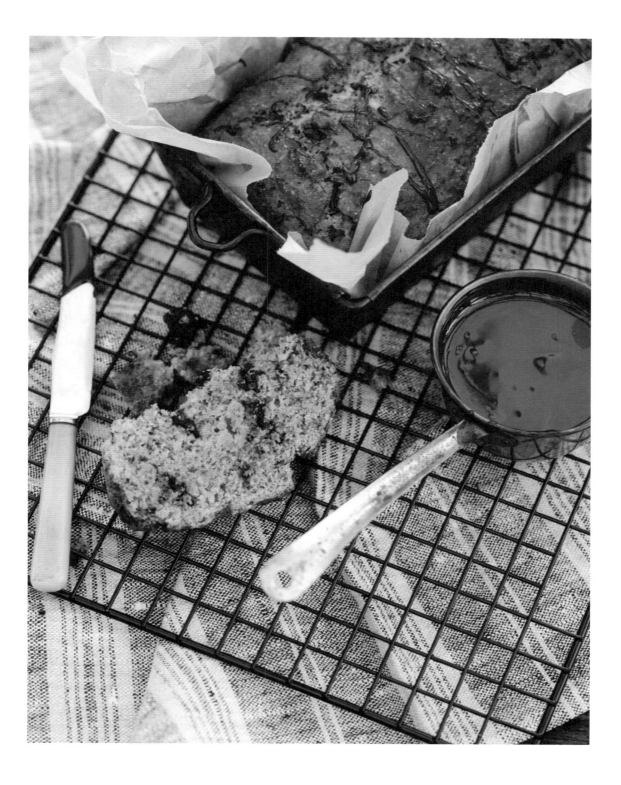

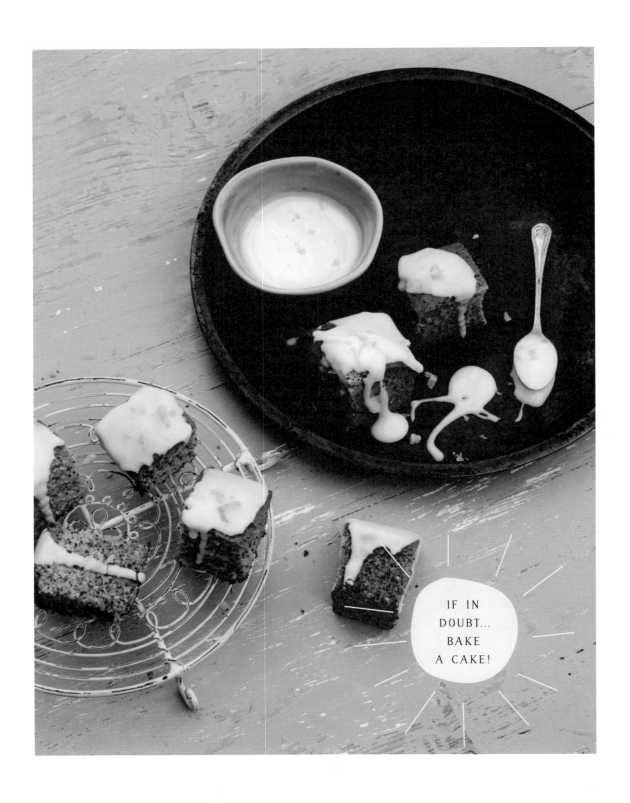

IF IN
DOUBT...
BAKE
A CAKE!

LEMON DRIZZLE & POPPY SEED SQUARES

Everyone needs one good baking recipe in their repertoire. And if I'm going to eat cake, I'd much rather bake it myself from scratch because I know exactly what is going in there and I can make it and enjoy it while it's fresh. I first made a version of this recipe in the kitchens of Dublin Cookery School and over time I've adapted it. These Lemon Drizzle & Poppy Seed Squares are an indulgence, but I love any excuse to make them.

○ ○

MAKES 16 SQUARES

For the cake

185ml warm milk
40g poppy seeds
185g unsalted butter, softened
220g caster sugar
3 eggs
300g self-raising flour
zest of 1 lemon

For the lemon icing

300g icing sugar
juice of 1 lemon

Preheat the oven to 150°C/300°F/gas 2. Grease an 18cm (7 inch) square tin and line it with parchment paper.

Mix the warm milk and poppy seeds in a small bowl or measuring jug and set aside for 15 minutes.

Whisk the butter and sugar together in a large bowl until pale and creamy. Add the eggs one at a time, whisking until the mixture is fluffy. Add the flour, the milk and poppy seed mixture, and the lemon zest, whisking after each addition. Whisk for about 5 minutes, until the batter is pale and thick.

Pour the batter into the prepared tin and bake for 50 minutes or until a skewer inserted comes out clean. If the cake is not golden-brown, increase the oven to 180°C/400°F/gas 4 and bake for a further 5 minutes. Set aside to cool for 10 minutes, then remove from the tin and leave to cool on a wire rack.

For the lemon icing, place the icing sugar and lemon juice in a bowl and mix well until smooth. Place the cooled cake on a board and cut into squares. Drizzle over the lemon icing and serve.

SWEET & STICKY PECANS

Nuts are full of nutritional goodness. My only problem with these Sweet & Sticky Pecans is that I want to eat them all at once. They're as versatile as they are yummy: perfect for a snack if people call to visit and also great scattered on salads throughout the week.

○ ○

MAKES A HANDFUL OF NUTS
a handful of pecans
2 tbsp agave syrup
a pinch of sea salt

Preheat the oven to 160°C/325°F/gas 3.

Spread the pecans on a large baking tin, drizzle over the agave syrup and sprinkle over the salt. Roast the pecans for about 20 minutes, turning once. Leave them to cool on the tray or serve them hot straight away.

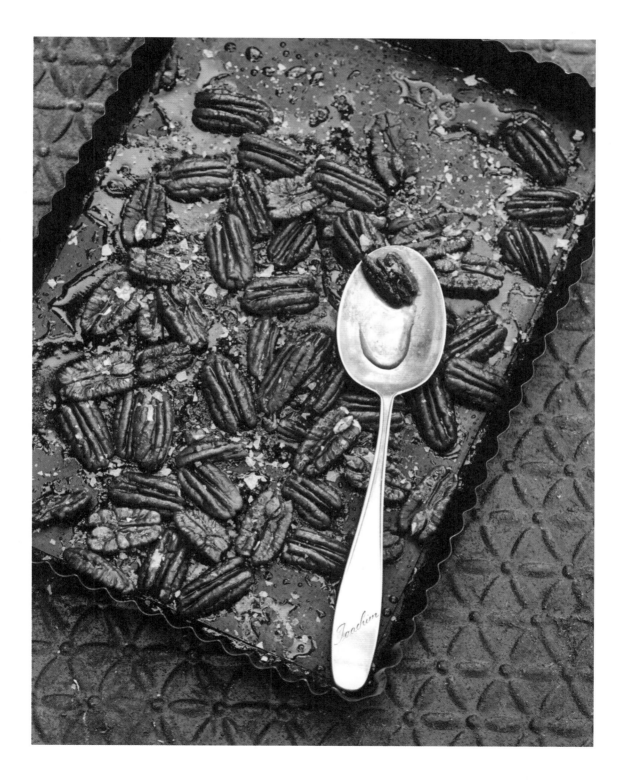

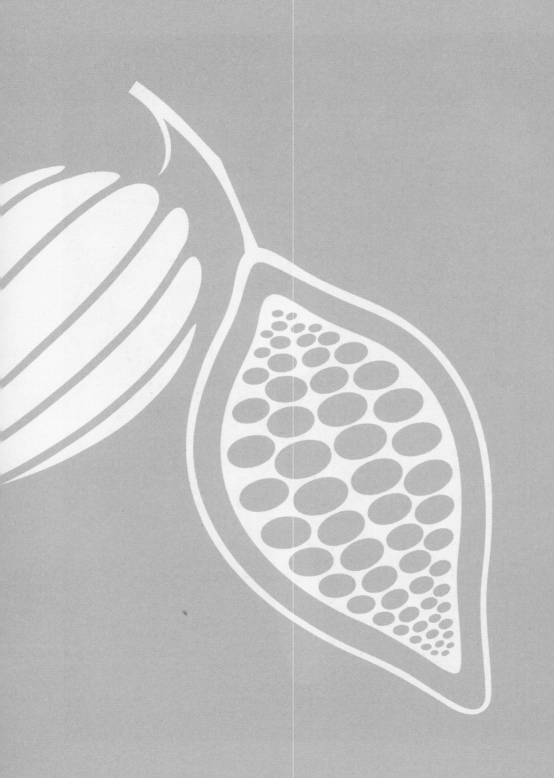

JAMIE HEASLIP'S BROWNIES

I love rugby and we are very fortunate in Ireland that our national players are incredibly good at what they do. Their approach is really professional and has brought with it bucket-loads of success in the past few years. Jamie Heaslip has been a massive part of Irish rugby success. He's had the honour of captaining Ireland and Leinster. It's fair to say that he's a bit of a sporting legend. And off the pitch, Jamie is involved in a beautiful Dublin restaurant called Bear. So what recipe did a rugby legend want to contribute to my book? A lovely gooey, chocolatey recipe for brownies! Just goes to show that even amazing rugby players need the occasional chocolate hit to keep them going.

° °

MAKES 6 BIG BROWNIES
(OR 12 MINI)
250g unsalted butter
200g dark chocolate (70% cocoa solids), chopped
4 eggs
350g caster sugar
80g cocoa powder
65g plain flour
1 tsp baking powder

Preheat the oven to 180°C/350°F/gas 4. Grease an 18cm (7 inch) square tin and line it with parchment paper.

Melt the butter and chocolate in a large heatproof bowl over a pan of simmering water and set aside to cool slightly.

Lightly whisk the eggs in a medium bowl.

Sift the sugar, cocoa powder, flour and baking powder into the melted chocolate mixture. Stir in the eggs and mix well.

Pour the mixture into the prepared tin and bake for about 30 minutes or until firm in the centre and a skewer inserted comes out clean. Remove from the oven and leave to cool, then cut into squares and serve.

STRAWBERRY TREATS

These are so tasty and easy to make – and they look pretty too. If you're having friends over for dinner you could make these in advance, since they store well in the fridge. And if it's a treat night, these go really well with a glass of wine.

○ ○ ○○

MAKES 6 TREATS

50g dark chocolate (70% cocoa solids), chopped

6 juicy strawberries

50g desiccated coconut

Melt the chocolate in a heatproof bowl over a pan of simmering water. Dip each strawberry into the melted chocolate and sprinkle over some desiccated coconut.

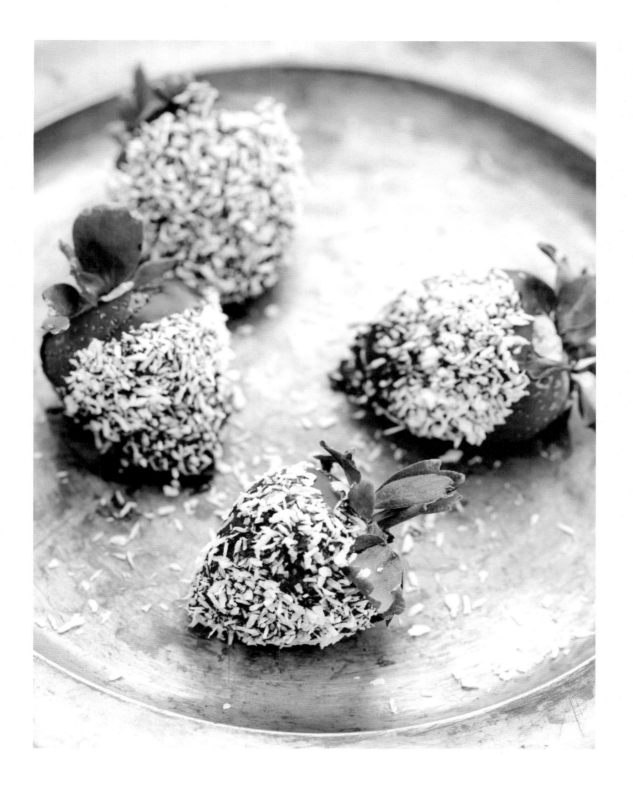

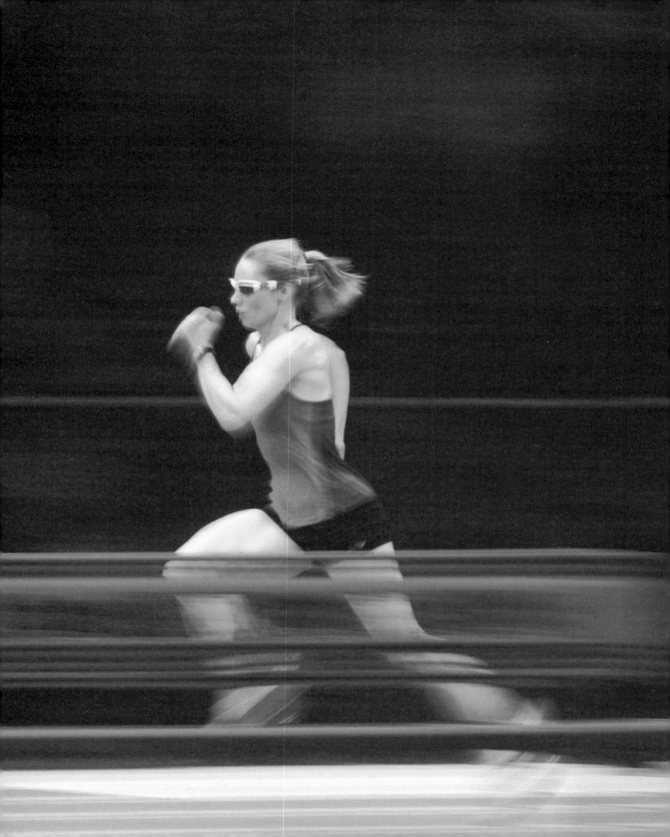

LIFE LESSONS
FROM THE 'OVAL OFFICE'

Being a full-time track athlete for a decade has taught me many lessons and they often pop into my head when I'm running around that big oval office.

1 Always CHOOSE GOOD PEOPLE TO WORK WITH. They are the people who you would choose to go to a desert island with.

2 Accept that YOU DON'T KNOW EVERYTHING. Not having the answers is not weakness; being unwilling to find the answers is.

3 DON'T TRY TO BE PERFECT – just try to be a little better all the time. Perfection is not an option. I never ran a perfect race.

4 BE CONFIDENT, not arrogant. It's easy to mix up these two things: at times, I certainly have.

5 Learn to HAVE BLINKERS. Relying on the opinions of others is too fickle a way to live.

6 LEARN NEW SKILLS no matter what age you are. I learned to swim at 32. Women in their eighties were faster than me!

7 DON'T BE SCARED to make the tougher choices:
'Two roads diverged in a wood, and I —
I took the one less traveled by,
And that has made all the difference.'

8 TAKE THE BLAME. It's easy to blame others when things don't work out but, ultimately, the buck stops with you. Man up, woman up, take the blame.

9 BLACK AND WHITE is hard to come by. Most of the time, things are quite grey with no exact right or exact wrong.

10 APPRECIATE LUCK. Every now and then you get a little at the right time.

QUICK CHOCCIE CHIP COOKIES

These cookies are really lovely and very easy to do. It is pure joy to have one warm out of the oven with a cup of hot tea. I love the simplicity of this recipe. There are just four ingredients, so there's really no excuse not to get baking.

MAKES 6 COOKIES

2 bananas, peeled and mashed

50g dark chocolate (70% cocoa solids), chopped

40g porridge oats

25g desiccated coconut

Preheat the oven to 160°C/325°F/gas 3. Line a large baking sheet with parchment paper.

Place all of the ingredients in a large bowl and use your hands to mix everything together. The bananas will bind the mixture so make sure to give them a good squeeze with your fingers. When the cookie dough has formed, roll it into balls and place them a few centimetres apart on the prepared baking sheet. Use your hands to flatten the cookies slightly.

Bake for 15 minutes. Allow the cookies to cool slightly on the tray before removing to a wire rack.

MANGO NUT BREAD

This bread is a little bit healthy and a little bit bold. It's full of lovely tropical flavours: mango, coconut and lime. It gives you a sugar-level boost so I only like to have it when I feel like I've earned it. Nothing tastes better than a slice of this after a really successful training session.

∘ ∘ ∘ ∘

MAKES 1 LOAF

½ ripe banana, peeled and mashed

½ ripe mango, peeled and diced

120g plain flour (I don't bother sifting –
  but that's just me)

60ml coconut oil, melted

6 tbsp brown sugar

4 tbsp agave syrup

2 tbsp flaked almonds

2 tbsp macadamia nuts, roughly chopped

2 tbsp pecan nuts, roughly chopped

1 egg

½ tsp bread soda (bicarbonate of soda)

a pinch of salt

juice of ½ lime

Preheat the oven to 190°C/375°F/gas 5. Grease a 900g (2lb) loaf tin and line it with parchment paper.

Mix all of the ingredients in a large bowl until just combined. Pour the batter into the prepared loaf tin. Bake for 45 minutes or until a skewer inserted comes out clean. Set aside to cool for 10 minutes, then remove from the tin and leave to cool on a wire rack.

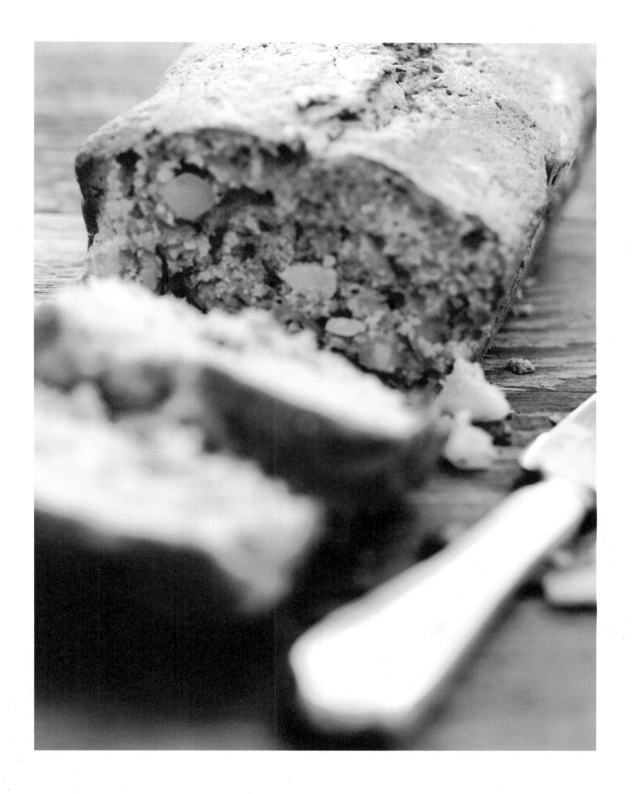

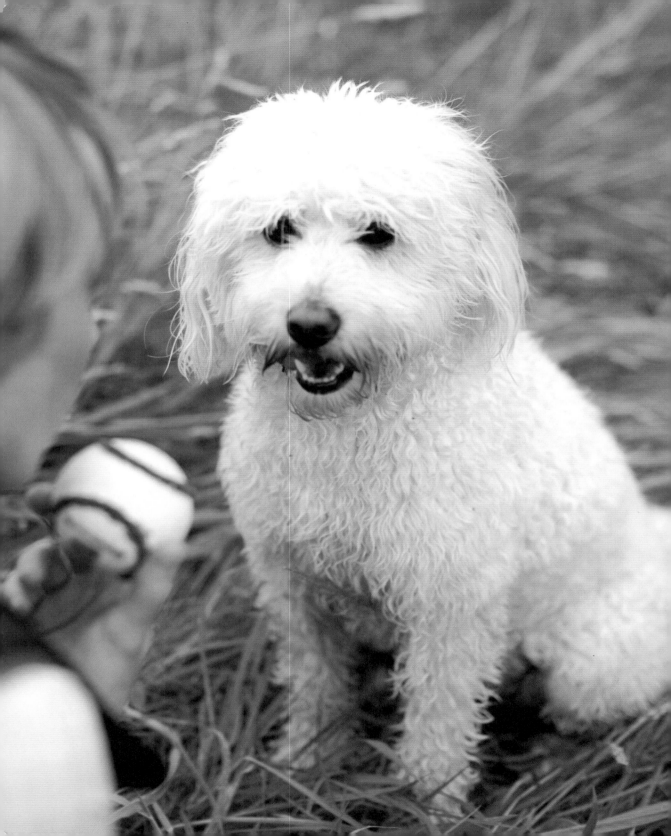

BERLINO'S ICY TREAT

Chances are that if you've heard about me, you've heard about my dog Berlino! She has a keen interest in track and sailing and she is a loyal training partner in all weathers. Even before we got Berlino, she was playing her part in improving my performance. Coming up to the 2009 World Outdoor Championships in Berlin, Peter and I made a serious bet. I'd wanted to get a dog for ages and Peter said that he would agree if I did two things at the Championships: come in Top 5 in my race and break the Irish record. At the time, I was racing badly and I was ranked well outside the Top 30 in the world. Peter wasn't that enthusiastic about us getting a dog, so I think he felt pretty confident in his bet. I kept my eyes on the prize, though. As the Championships approached, I started running faster in training and feeling really well. When it came to the crunch, I ran my race and won my bet. I finished fourth and I broke the Irish record! As I came off the track I spoke to the press. They wanted me to give the usual analysis of the race, when all I wanted to talk about was getting a dog! Berlino was named after the mascot of the Championships. As it turned out, Peter was very happy to lose that bet – and Berlino moved in with us.

Here is a recipe I make for the furry boss. I believe that every athlete, human or canine, needs a treat now and then.

MAKES 2 ICE CUBE TRAYS
350ml chicken or beef stock, simmering
a few slices of cooked chicken or beef, finely chopped
50g premium nutrition dog food, such as Royal Canin

Place all of the ingredients in a medium bowl and leave to cool. Pour the mixture into an ice cube tray, store in the freezer and serve as needed.

I've written the recipes in this book using the metric system but I sometimes find it handy to cook using measuring cups and spoons. For any readers who would like to cook this way, here is a conversion chart of common ingredients. Some of these conversions have been rounded up or down for the sake of convenience.

CONVERSION
CHART